# How to set up an Acute Stroke Service

Iris Q. Grunwald • Klaus Fassbender
Ajay K. Wakhloo

# How to set up an Acute Stroke Service

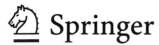 Springer

Prof. Iris Q. Grunwald
Acute Vascular Imaging Centre
Oxford University Hospitals NHS Trust
and NIHR Biomedical Research Centre
Headley Way
Oxford OX3 9DU
UK

Prof. Dr. Klaus Fassbender
Department of Neurology
Saarland University
Kirrberger Strasse
66421 Homburg
Germany

Prof. Ajay K. Wakhloo
Department of Radiology
Division of Neuroimaging & Intervention NII
University of Massachusetts
Lake Avenue N. 55
Worcester, MA 01655
USA

Illustrations: Jean-Philippe Legrand "Aster"
www.dessindepresse.com and www.cartoonevent.com

Medical graphic design: Eloise White
www.eloisewhite-illustrator.com

ISBN 978-3-642-21404-2          e-ISBN 978-3-642-21405-9
DOI 10.1007/978-3-642-21405-9
Springer Heidelberg Dordrecht London New York

Library of Congress Control Number: 2011942220

Springer is part of Springer Science+Business Media (www.springer.com)

# Foreword

Setting up something new is often challenging, particularly if it involves changing the existing routine that people have become used to. The challenges can be particularly daunting when it comes to developing a new clinical service in a modern health care system. This is rarely more so than in setting up an acute stroke service. However, this book provides clinicians and managers with all of the information they need to plan for and overcome the foreseeable obstacles to setting up a new service as well as providing a blueprint for a highly effective service.

The book assumes little prior knowledge about acute stroke and provides all of the relevant background information necessary to understand the most important issues, including summaries of the evidence supporting each of the main clinical interventions that currently make up an acute stroke service. The "how-to-do-it" style of the book is testimony to the fact that the authors have themselves set up services and are all highly experienced in the practical delivery of acute stroke care.

The coverage of the important issues relating to each stage of the patient pathway is particularly valuable, as is the emphasis on the practical problems to be overcome in areas such as pre-hospital care and the imaging pathway. Coverage of other key considerations in setting up a new service, including space, staffing, teams, budget and management, is also extremely useful. There are, in fact, no major issues that are not covered.

I am certain this manual will prove invaluable to anybody who wishes to either improve an existing stroke service or to set up a new service from scratch.

Professor of Clinical Neurology                                    Peter M. Rothwell
University of Oxford

# Preface

The authors have made every effort in preparing this book to provide accurate and up-to-date information, which is in accordance with accepted clinical practice at the time of publication. However, the authors, editors and publishers can make no guarantees that the information contained in this book is totally free from error, not least because clinical standards vary in different countries and are subject to constant change through research and regulation. The authors, editors and publishers therefore disclaim all liability for direct or consequential damages resulting from the use of material contained in this publication. We strongly advised readers to pay careful attention to information provided by their regulatory department and manufacturer of drugs or equipment they plan to use.

Every dosage schedule or every form of application described is entirely at the user's own risk and responsibility. Some drugs and medial devices presented in the book do not have or have only limited Food and Drug Administration (FDA) clearance for use in restricted research settings. It is the responsibility of the user to ascertain the regulatory status of each drug and advice planned for use. The authors, editors and publishers have taken care to confirm the accuracy of the information presented but are not responsible for errors or omissions or for any consequences from application of the information provided in this book. They take no warranty, expressed or implied, with respect to the information provided and the application of the information remains the responsibility of the practitioner. In view of ongoing research, changes in Government regulations, and the constant flow of information, the reader is urged to double check applicability of the content.

# About This Book

Because you are reading this book, I presume that you have been asked or are involved in the challenging task of setting up or optimizing an acute stroke service. For this you are going to need a basic insight into the current treatment of stroke.

You might ask yourself, why is the topic of acute ischemic stroke of such great interest today? The answer is simple:

- *Stroke represents a major economic health burden, and nowadays is treatable.*

Historically, stroke treatment consisted of prevention and rehabilitation – but successful options in acute stroke treatment have dramatically increased. Administration of i.v.-lytics as well as endovascular stroke treatment has been shown highly beneficial in clinical trials and effective in net cost savings. Also, developments in CT and MR imaging and the availability of effective mechanical stroke devices offer the prospect of improvements in diagnosis, treatment, and outcome.

However, time is of the essence in the management of stroke, and we are called upon to take measures to ensure that the response to acute stroke is both rapid and effective.

This book aims to give an insight into the recent changes regarding acute ischemic stroke management where treatment of acute stroke can now begin during the pre-hospital phase, before a stroke physician is even involved. No matter if you are the one that has taken on the challenge of setting up an acute stroke service or whether you just want to familiarize yourself with current management options, this book offers a concise and practical guide on how to set up and efficiently run an acute stroke service. It provides the essential knowledge on current imaging and treatment options and helps organize a site-specific stroke pathway to treat patients as quickly as possible in order to optimize the benefit to the patient as well as to maximize the cost-effectiveness.

This book uses modern project management techniques to provide guidance in setting up a stroke service, but more importantly gives you the essential knowledge to make such a concept work. It also aims to provide tools to conquer the multiple technical and administrative challenges you will face.

We include a short overview of relevant, clinical trials carried out to date and describe different treatment options for acute stroke. The challenging, multidisciplinary nature of care and the importance of pre- and post-hospital management are emphasized.

Each chapter is self-contained, so you can read the chapters that are most relevant to you first. However, if you do not have any previous knowledge of the medical condition "ischemic stroke" and are unfamiliar with essential diagnostic and current treatment options, you should take the time to read those chapters that explain current stroke diagnosis and management options.

## Icons Used in This Book

Although the icons are pretty standard and self-explanatory here is a brief explanation of what they mean:

 TIPs suggest alternatives or advice

 Key points point out important information you want to keep in mind

 Studies or extra background information

 Example

 This icon invites you to take your own notes

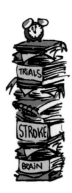 References and further reading

# Acknowledgement

We would like to express our gratitude to the publishers Springer. Special thanks go to Ute Heilmann, Meike Stoeck, Wilma McHugh and Karthikeyan Gurunathan. Also we are grateful for the support of the NIHR Biomedical Research Centre, Oxford, the UK Stroke Research Network and all our friends who have helped in the creation of this book.

# Contents

# Definitions and Abbreviations

| | |
|---|---|
| ADC | Apparent diffusion coefficients |
| AHA | American Heart Association |
| AIS | acute ischemic stroke |
| AP | anterior-posterior |
| Aphasia | difficulty in language production and/or understanding |
| Apoplexy | different name for stroke |
| ASA | American Stroke Association |
| BAC | Brain Attack Coalition |
| BI | Barthel Index |
| BONnet | intracranial flow restoration device |
| Brain attack | describes the typical features of stroke |
| Brain hemorrhage | blood that has burst out into the brain |
| Cerebral infarction | death of brain tissue |
| Cerebral thrombosis | clot in the blood vessel of the brain |
| Circle of Willis | connection of the arteries supplying the brain |
| CA | California |
| CI | confidence interval, contra indication |
| CL | centralized laboratory |
| CNS | central nervous system |
| CRC | mechanical recanalization device |
| CRUK | Cancer Research United Kingdom |
| CSF | cerebrospinal fluid |
| CT | computed tomography |
| CTA | computed tomography angiography |
| CTP | computed tomography perfusion |
| DECIMAL | DEcompressive Craniectomy In MALignant middle cerebral artery infarction |
| DESTINY | DEcompressive Surgery for the Treatment of malignant INfarction of the middle cerebral arterY |
| Dissection | internal splitting of the vessel wall |
| DSA | digital subtraction angiography |
| Dyna-CT | innovative system for 3-dimensional reconstruction |
| DWI | diffusion weighted imaging |

| | |
|---|---|
| DW-MRI | diffusion-weighted MRI sequence that can detect an ischemic stroke within minutes |
| Dysphagia | difficulty to swallow |
| ECA | external carotid artery |
| ECASS III | placebo controlled trial of rtPA in acute ischemic stroke where thrombolysis is initiated between 3 and 4 hours after stroke onset |
| ED | Emergency Department |
| Edema | swelling of the brain |
| EFNS | European Federation of Neurological Societies |
| EKOS | mechanical recanalization device |
| Embolus | blood clot within the vessel |
| EMS | Emergency Medical Services |
| Epidemiology | incidence, distribution and control of disease in a population |
| ESO | European Stroke Organization |
| EST | endovascular stroke treatment |
| FDA | Food and Drug Administration |
| FLAIR | Fluid-attenuated inversion recovery MRI |
| GCS | Glasgow Coma Scale |
| G-DRG | German Diagnosis Related Groups |
| GOS | Glasgow Outcome Scale |
| GP | General Practitioner |
| h | hour |
| HAMLET | study looking at efficacy of decompressive surgery |
| Hemiparesis | paralysis of the face, arm and or leg on one side of the body |
| Hemorrhagic transformation | bleeding into the brain that occurs after the cerebral infarct |
| Hypertension | high blood pressure |
| Hypotension | low blood pressure |
| ICA | internal carotid artery |
| ICD | International Classification of Diseases |
| ICH | intra-cerebral hemorrhage |
| ICU | intensive care unit |
| IMS II/III | stroke trials |
| Incidence of stroke | number of strokes per year |
| INR | Interventional Neuroradiology |
| Ischemic stroke | stroke caused by loss of blood supply to the brain |
| i.a. | intra-arterial |
| IT-expert | Information Technology expert |
| i.v. | intra-vanous |
| Lacunar infarction | a stroke caused by blockage of end arteries that will eventually leave a small hole called lacunar |
| MCA | middle cerebral artery |

| | |
|---|---|
| MELT | Middle cerebral artery Embolism Local fibrinolytic interventional Trial |
| MERCI | mechanical recanalization device |
| MN | Minnesota |
| MRA | magnetic resonance angiography |
| MRI | magnetic resonance imaging |
| mRS | modified Rankin Scale |
| mMTT | medium Mean Transit Time |
| Multimodal imaging | combining imaging techniques |
| MVO | multiple vessel occlusion |
| Myocardial infarct | heart attack |
| n | number of patients |
| Neurons | brain cells |
| NHS | National Health Service |
| NICE | National Institute for Health and Clinical Excellence |
| NIHSS | National Institute of Health Stroke Scale |
| NINDS | National Institute of Neurologic Disease |
| NNT | number needed to treat |
| NSA | National Stroke Association |
| NY | New York |
| Occlusion | blockage of the vessel |
| off-label | use does not match the instructions for use |
| OPS | Operation and Procedure Key for medical reimbursement |
| OR | odds ratio |
| PbR | Payment by Result |
| PCA | posterior cerebral artery |
| pCR | phenox Clot Retriever |
| PHENOX | mechanical recanalization device |
| Penumbra-System | mechanical recanalization device |
| Penumbra | Salvageable brain tissue |
| PICA | posterior inferior cerebellar artery |
| POC | Point-of-Care |
| PROACT 2 | PROlyse in Acute cerebral Thromboembolism 2, randomized clinical trial using i.a. urokinase in acute MCA stroke |
| PT/INR | prothrombin time (international normalized ratio) |
| PWI | perfusion weighted imaging |
| rCBV | regional cerebral blood volume |
| RR | relative risk |
| rtPA | recombinant tissue plasminogen activator |
| SAH | subarachnoid hemorrhage, a bleed that occurs in the brain |
| Secondary stroke prevention | prevention of a subsequent stroke |
| SOP | Standard Operating Procedures |

| | |
|---|---|
| Spasticity | the tone of the muscles is increased. This can result in contractions |
| SU | Stroke Unit |
| T2* MRI | T2 star weighted magnetic resonance imaging |
| tPA | tissue plasminogen activator |
| Thrombolysis | breaking up a blood clot with medication |
| TIA | transient ischemic attack with symptoms lasting for less than 24 hours |
| TICI | Thrombolysis In Cerebral Infarction |
| TIMI | Thrombolysis In Myocardial Infarction, a scoring system from 0 to 3 |
| UK | United Kingdom |
| Urokinase | thrombolytic agent |
| US | United States |
| USA | United States of America |
| WA | Washington |
| WBS | Work Breakdown Structure |
| WHO | World Health Organization |

# About the Authors

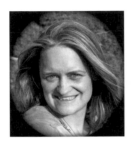 Prof. Iris Quasar Grunwald studied Medicine in Germany and did her residency training in Neurology and Radiology. She obtained her PhD in Radiology and Neuroradiology and a Diploma in Health Economics and Hospital Management. Prof. Grunwald has published more than 90 peer-reviewed articles and several book chapters, mainly in the field of neurointervention. She has specific expertise in procedures such as intracerebral intra-arterial fibrinolysis and thrombectomy for emergency stroke therapy and intracranial angioplasty and stenting.

Prof. Grunwald has an international reputation in implementing acute stroke interventions and has been involved with research projects related to building and enabling acute stroke interventions regionally within the Saarland, nationally within Germany as well as internationally as European Principal Investigator in international clinical trials related to revascularization in acute stroke. In addition she has conducted several lecture tours to leading US clinical stroke centers on the subjects of acute stroke intervention and management. In February 2009 she transferred to the UK, Oxford University Hospitals, to run the interventional stroke service within the Acute Vascular Imaging Centre, from where she leads her international trials.

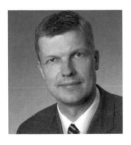 Prof. Klaus Fassbender possesses a broad scientific and clinical expertise in neurology and stroke medicine. He worked at the Department of internal medicine, Basel, Switzerland (1989–1990), and Max-Planck Institute for Psychiatry, Munich (1991–1992), and became involved in acute stroke research i.e., at the Department of Neurology Mannheim University of Heidelberg (chair: Prof. M. Hennerici) (1992–2002). After his stay at the Department of Neurology Goettingen (2002–2004), he became chairman of the Department of Neurology, Saarland University in 2005.

Currently, the focus of research of the Department of Neurology of Saarland University is the elaboration of optimal stroke management, e.g., by accelerating door-to-needle times by a novel pathway that includes diagnosis (incl. point-of-care laboratory) and causal treatment of stroke at a single site ("stroke room") or by first establishment of a "Mobile Stroke Unit" for pre-hospital stroke treatment. He was vice president of his University in 2007-2009, published more than 100 peer-reviewed articles and contributed to major national neurological guidelines.

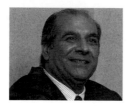 Prof. Ajay K. Wakhloo, a board certified Radiologist and Neuroradiologist specialized in Neuroendovascular surgery has made innovative contributions to the field of endovascular surgical treatment of brain aneurysms, brain arteriovenous shunts and stroke. Dr. Wakhloo is the Director of Neurointerventional Radiology/Endovascular Neurosurgery and the Director of Clinical Research in the Department of Radiology at the University of Massachusetts Medical School, and Co-Director of the New England Center for Stroke Research. He has served as Principle or Co-Investigator on grants from industry, private foundations and the National Institutes of Health. His research has led to discoveries that have produced several patents and has received numerous awards, including the Best Doctors in America 2005–2012. Dr. Wakhloo completed his doctorate of medicine at the University of Mainz, Germany in 1984, where he also received his doctorate of philosophy in the study of metabolic disorders. He received his habilitation in 1996 at the University of Tuebingen, Germany following the publications and presentation of his novel research about the effect of stent- induced flow remodeling to treat intracranial aneurysms. Dr. Wakhloo has published more than 150 papers in peer-reviewed journals and books and is the editor of the book Thrombus and Stroke, published in 2008.

**With contributions by:**

**Marianne Davidson-Beker** BA, P.G.Dip. Tch.&Learn, MPS has over 25 years' experience in a business management role and was the business manager of the Experimental Medicine Division, Nuffield Department of Clinical Medicine, University of Oxford, UK.

**Birgit Bock** has spent over 15 years as Director of Clinical Trials for an international Clinical Research Organization, overseeing regulatory affairs as well as clinical trials. She lives in Paris, from where she consults to international companies for CE-marking studies, and clinical trials in Europe to support US FDA 510(k) or PMA requirements.

**Dr. Anna Luisa Kühn´s** research interest lies within interventional neuroradiology. She has authored numerous publications in this field. She is working in the New England Center for Stroke Research, Department of Radiology, University of Massachusetts Medical School, MA, USA.

# Part I

# Understanding Your Goals:
# The What, Why and Who

# Essential Basics

## 1.1    What Is Stroke?

"Stroke" is a sudden loss of brain function caused by disruption of the blood flow to the brain. This can happen due to an occluded blood vessel (acute ischemic stroke) or rupture of a blood vessel (hemorrhagic stroke), which causes a bleed (Fig. 1.1).

This book is focused on defining and describing the treatment strategies for the medical condition of "acute ischemic stroke," when a sudden occlusion of an intracranial blood vessel causes an acute onset of symptoms. These symptoms can include numbness or weakness in the face, arm, or leg, difficulty in speaking or understanding, sudden dizziness, blurred or loss of vision in one or even both eyes, loss of balance, difficulty swallowing, headache, confusion, and unconsciousness.

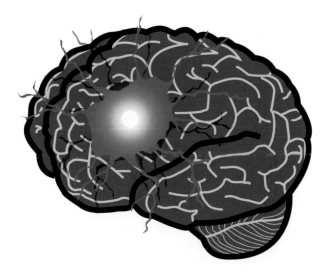

**Fig. 1.1** "Stroke" is a sudden loss of brain function

I.Q. Grunwald et al., *How to set up an Acute Stroke Service*, DOI 10.1007/978-3-642-21405-9_1, © Springer-Verlag Berlin Heidelberg 2012

In addition, a wider range of cognitive/neurobehavioral deficits has recently been attributed to stroke. These are apraxia, memory loss and dementia, as well as depression and other psychiatric disorders.

If stroke symptoms do not cause permanent brain damage but resolve within 24 h, they are called transient ischemic attacks (TIA). They cause the same symptoms as a stroke and are an important warning sign that a stroke may be imminent. Very recently, this term is more and more criticized as novel imaging methods often reveal ischemic cerebral damage despite disappearance of symptoms within 24 h, arguing for a real stroke rather than an only transient functional disorder. A TIA with positive imaging signs of brain infarction represents an extremely unstable condition with a high, imminent risk of stroke.

## 1.2    What Happens During a Stroke?

The occlusion of an artery in the neck or in the brain deprives a section of the brain of its nutrients such as glucose and oxygen. The occlusion of the artery is most commonly caused by thrombus that has travelled (embolized) to the brain. This thrombus can come from the heart or from plaque in a more proximal artery. Other causes can be intracranial stenosis caused by atherosclerosis or infectious disease (Fig. 1.2).

## 1.3    Why Set Up a Stroke Service?

There are many reasons for setting up an acute stroke service. Next to offering optimized treatment and complying with current guidelines and recommendations (Chap. 2), one of the main reasons is to reduce the economic burden of stroke, which constitutes a major claim on our health care budgets worldwide. Also, with an increased life expectancy, the incidence of stroke is continuously rising. On the other hand, stroke awareness among the general public is still lacking.

Stroke Statistic Information from the US National Stroke Association showed that in adults over the age of 50:
- 38% did not know where a stroke occurs.
- Only 1% could name stroke as a leading cause of death.
- 40% did not know any warning signs.
- 12% did not know any risk factors.
- 50% did not know when strokes occur.
- Only 40% would call an emergency number when they experienced stroke like symptoms.
(Stroke Statistic Information from National Stroke Association: www.stroke.org/Stroke_Facts.html)

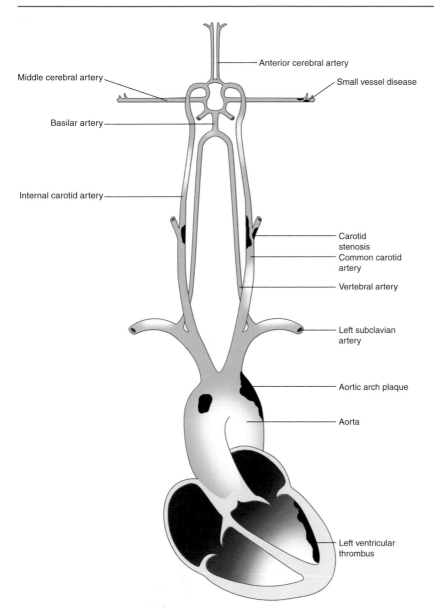

**Fig. 1.2** The common causes of acute ischemic stroke are thrombus from the left ventricle, cardiogenic emboli, or thrombus caused by carotid stenosis or dissection. Adapted from Rymer, & Silverman, (2009). Ischemic Stroke: An Atlas of Investigation and Treatment (1st ed. p. 3). Clinical Pub

Public education about stroke is thus important, and due to increased preventative medicine education, public awareness is now gradually increasing.

It has been shown that by organizing stroke care in a stroke service, significantly better health outcomes can be achieved – with the same budget (Huijsman et al. 2001).

**1**

Integrating public education, correct dispatch, pre-hospital diagnosis and triage, hospital stroke system development, and stroke unit management as well as rehabilitation will inevitably lead to significant improvements in stroke care.

### 1.3.1   To Address the Economic Burden of Stroke

Worldwide, 15 million people suffer a stroke each year. About five million of these patients will die; another five million will survive with permanent disability (UN Chronicle Health Watch 2005). It is estimated that at 1 year follow-up, 30% of the stroke patients will have died, and 40% will be dependent on family or caregivers for acts of daily living (Warlow et al. 2001).

In the USA, every 40 seconds a patient will suffer a stroke. Each day there are more than 2,000 new strokes, and each year there are more than 750,000 new strokes. Stroke is the third leading cause of death in the USA and the leading cause of adult disability. There are more than 4.4 million stroke survivors with disability.

The prognosis of stroke is poor with a 30–35% incidence of death and a 35–40% incidence of major disability. Of those who survive a stroke, approximately 10–18% will have another stroke within 1 year.

Of those patients who suffer a stroke:
- 31% require assistance with care.
- 20% need help with walking.
- 16% are institutionalized.
- 71% are vocationally impaired after 7 years.
- 35% are unemployable below 65 years.
(Framingham Study Cohort 1991).

The health care cost associated with stroke is more than US$ 50 billion (direct cost more than US$ 30 billion and US$ 20 billion indirect cost).

This makes stroke a major disease in both medical and economic terms, placing a considerable strain on patients, payers and society regarding premature death, long-term disability, restricted social functioning, cost of care, and informal caregiver time (Caro et al. 2000).

The financial burden of stroke is likely to rise even further, given that the number of elderly people is expected to increase in industrialized countries – where stroke is already the third most common cause of death.

In developing countries, as death from infectious diseases and malnutrition declines, stroke incidence rises due to decreased physical activity and dietary changes. Sixty percent of all strokes occur in low- and middle-income countries, and it is expected that by 2040, a billion adults aged 65 years or older will be at risk of stroke (Reddy and Yusuf 1998).

Regarding cost, the most contributing factors during the first year are institutional costs such as acute hospitalization, rehabilitation, and nursing home care. Patients that die shortly after a stroke accumulate significantly less total costs; on the other hand, the costs per day alive are significantly higher.

The long-term cost of a patient's first ischemic stroke is estimated at US$159.000 for a stroke resulting in major impairment, and $58.600 for a stroke resulting in minor impairment (Caro and Huybrechts 1999). The high cost comprises of hospitalization rates, expensive in-hospital treatment, and high rates of long-term disability in the survivors.

The Erlangen stroke project estimated the overall cost per patient that survives after a first ischemic stroke for a time period of 5 years to be € 18.517. The discounted lifetime cost per case was € 43.129. National projections for the period 2006–2025 estimated national direct ischemic stroke costs of € 108.6 billion in Germany alone (The Erlangen stroke project 2006).

About one million first ischemic strokes are estimated to occur each year in the *European Union*.

In *England, Wales, and Scotland*, stroke alone accounts for 3–4% of the direct cost of healthcare that includes hospitalization, rehabilitation, medical treatment, and long-term care (Isard and Forbes 1992). In England, stroke costs the economy around £7 billion annually. This comprises direct costs to the National Health Service of £2.8 billion, costs of informal care of £2.4 billion, and costs because of lost productivity and disability of £1.8 billion (Mant et al. 2004).

*In the USA*, stroke remains the third leading cause of death. The USA has between 4 and 5 million residents affected by stroke, which constitutes an US incidence rate of 600,000–700,000 per year and contributes to 150,000 US deaths annually.

If the proportion of all ischemic stroke patients that receive tPA were increased to 20%, the realized cost savings would be approximately US$74 million respectively (Bogousslavsky and Paciaroni 2009).

*In Canada*, stroke is the leading cause of adult neurologic disability, which costs the Canadian economy at least $3 billion annually. Every year, more than 50,000 Canadians experience a stroke and more than 300,000 live with the ongoing effects (Heart and Stroke Foundation of Canada 2003).

*In the Netherlands*, stroke was estimated to be responsible for 3.2% of total health care costs in 1994, and 7.3% of the population were aged 75 and over (Evers et al. 2002).

The *Australian* Rural Health & Education Foundation reported that around 53,000 stroke events occur annually among Australians.

In 2004, around 220,000 Australians were living with stroke. The National Stroke Foundation in 2009 reported that strokes cost Australia an estimated $2.14 billion a year (Cadilhac et al. 2005).

The World Health Organization (WHO) estimated a stroke mortality rate of 280 per 100,000 people in *Russia* and 156 per 100,000 people in the *Ukraine* in 2002. The latter observation was on par with the stroke mortality rate reported in *China* and *Malawi* in 2002 (Bernard et al. 2003).

## 1.3.2   To Meet with Current Requirements

Over the past decade, stroke has been identified as a preventable and treatable disease. A functioning stroke service is not only clinically beneficial but it is able to generate hospital income while reducing total health care costs. This, and the growing awareness of the lack of diagnosis and treatment of patients that would potentially benefit from early stroke intervention, has increased the pressure many governments are now putting on the health care providers. The National Sentinel Audit figures for 2008 indicated that only 29% of stroke patients in England and Wales were able to access stroke unit care on the day of their stroke and only a minority of those eligible for thrombolytic treatment received it (National Sentinel Stroke Audit 2008). Increased stroke education has produced significant strides in public awareness, leading to a rising number of patients that arrive in the narrow, therapeutic time window – but also leading to increased pressure to provide stroke care in accordance with current national and international guidelines and recommendations.

## 1.3.3   To Efficiently Manage Stroke as a Potentially Treatable Disease

Over a decade ago, on June 18, 1996, the US Food and Drug Administration (FDA) approved the use of an intravenous lytic, namely, tissue plasminogen activator (tPA) as a therapy for acute ischemic stroke within 3 hours from onset. Since then the time window was expanded to 4.5 hours and intra-arterial lysis as well as mechanical stroke devices, that can target the clot directly in the brain, have been shown effective in early stroke treatment. However, across the world, only a fraction of the stroke patient population receives optimized treatment, with percentages ranging from 2% to 3% in the USA and 4% in Europe (Kleindorfer et al. 2008). Thus, the current treatment for most patients with acute ischemic stroke is limited to the management of the symptoms, antiplatelet therapy, secondary stroke prevention and rehabilitation. The reasons for non-treatment are varied but are often due to time constraints, inefficient workflow, and lack of knowledge about the course of the disease as well as current treatment options. The creation of stroke centers that offer thrombolysis and/or mechanical recanalization, therapy of complications, as well as secondary stroke prevention has been shown to improve overall stroke care.

With a structured stroke pathway that can include web-based tele-stroke programs and telemedicine, the lilliputian number of patients that currently receive stroke treatment can be dramatically increased, by focusing on restoring or improving perfusion to the ischemic area during the early moments after stroke, when intervention can make a profound difference to long-term outcome. Effective, timely stroke management and treatment, whether in hospital or in the community, is best undertaken by a specialized team. The time-sensitive nature of stroke can also necessitate local partnerships between academic medical centers and community hospitals, even in densely populated metropolitan centers. A pre-established emergency chain that is tailored toward the patients needs from onset of stroke symptoms to diagnosis and treatment can best reduce time delays and secure an efficient treatment of this so often devastating disease.

## 1.4    Understanding the Penumbra Concept

### 1.4.1    What Is the Penumbra?

The neuronal function depends on a sufficient oxygen and glucose supply. To supply the brain with these and other nutrients, an adequate cerebral blood flow (CBF) is essential. Any interruption of the blood supply will quickly result in neuronal dysfunction, which is then followed by irreversible damage.

> In human adults, the brain weighs approximately 1,400 g and represents only about 2% of the total body weight. However, it uses about 25% of total body oxygen and glucose per minute (Nagahiro et al. 1998).

*Example*
An occlusion of the left middle cerebral artery (MCA) (Fig. 1.3) would result in an irreversibly damaged ischemic core (black) of tissue with no or minimal cerebral blood flow. It would be surrounded by a potentially salvageable, slightly better perfused area (due to collateral circulation) which is called "penumbra" (orange).

The necessary cerebral blood flow for unimpaired brain function is normally about 50-ml/100 g brain/min (Fig. 1.4). The threshold for neuronal and

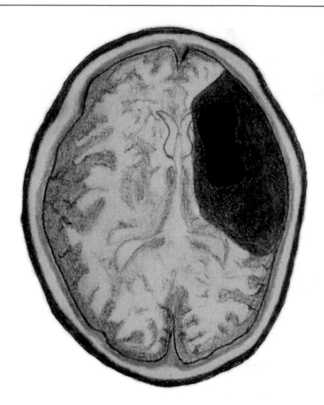

**Fig. 1.3** This figure shows the penumbra: the core (*black*) represents the center of severe ischemia with irreversible damage from where infarction develops rapidly. The penumbra (*orange*) is the marginally perfused area surrounding the core, which has the capacity to recover should perfusion be restored promptly

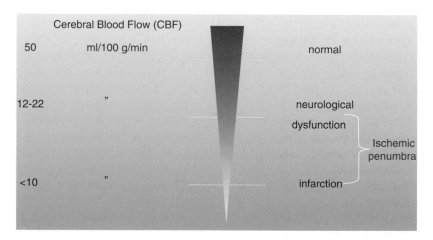

**Fig. 1.4** Thresholds for neuronal and electrical dysfunction

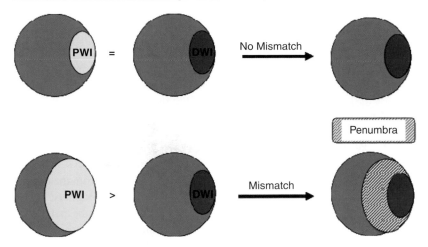

**Fig. 1.5** The penumbra is the ischemic region of under-perfused brain tissue that is metabolically impaired, electrically non-functioning but on a cellular basis is intact and still salvageable. This penumbra area is the target of acute stroke therapies and forms the basis for therapeutic interventions

electrical dysfunction lies at 12–22 ml/100 g/min. If this is not met, the electrical activity will cease. Although unable to function at these low perfusion levels, the cerebral tissue in the penumbra can recover unless the blood flow decreases below 10–12 ml/100 g/min (Heiss 2010; Branston et al. 1979).

The penumbra concept and the progression of irreversible damage are essential for the understanding of the pathophysiology of ischemic stroke. A simple definition of the penumbra would be "ischemic tissue that is potentially at risk for infarction but not yet irreversibly harmed."

The idea is that there are two ischemic thresholds in the development of cerebral infarction, one for reversible functional impairment and the other for irreversible morphological damage. Between these ranges is the penumbra (Fig. 1.5).

Information on the penumbra is most critical in the acute phase of stroke because not all the tissues supplied by the occluded artery will be affected simultaneously.

Usually, the more peripheral parts of the affected tissue will, at least for a short time, be able to maintain a minimum amount of its energy requirements – for example, through collateral flow.

Occasionally, spontaneous collateral reperfusion allows morphologic integrity of the penumbra to be preserved. Also, there is a variability in the functional thresholds of individual neurons, even within small cortical sectors, which explains the gradual development of neurological deficits. Whereas neuronal function is immediately impaired as flow declines below the threshold, the subsequent irreversible morphological damage is time dependent.

After cessation of the blood flow to a cerebral artery:
- The suppression of the electrical activity already occurs within 12–15 s.
- Inhibition of trans-synaptic excitation occurs after 2–4 min.
- The inhibition of electrical excitability takes place after only 4–6 min.
- Shortly thereafter the breakdown of the metabolism occurs.

## 1.4.2   Why Is the Penumbra Important?

After a stroke, the irreversible damage progresses over time from the core of the infarct center with the most severe flow reduction to the periphery, where the perfusion is less disturbed. Recovery of blood flow to the penumbra plays the central role in all therapeutic interventions.

The discrimination between infarct core and surrounding, potentially salvageable tissue is used for better identification of patients that might still benefit from treatment, either with rtPA or mechanical thrombectomy.

Recombinant tissue plasminogen activator (rtPA) is the only approved drug for acute stroke that has shown significant benefits when administered intravenously within the 4.5-h time window (ECASS III). However, the instructions for use (Boehringer) still refer to the previously accepted time window of 3 h and have not yet been amended, resulting in "off-label" use of this drug beyond the 3-h time window. Even with the expanded "off-label use," it is, unfortunately, often impossible to determine the onset of stroke (e.g., if the stroke happened during sleep), and thus, many patients cannot be treated because it is not known if they are within the approved time window when they present. Also, because of lack of adequate knowledge of the symptoms or due to poor response by health care providers, a large proportion of patients that might potentially benefit from recanalization are still admitted or processed for treatment too late.

Thus, over the last few years, much effort has been placed in the development of reliable imaging techniques to identify ischemic penumbra.

The identification of the penumbra can allow for selective rtPA use in those patients with a large penumbra and a small infarct core even beyond the 4.5-h time window, where it has been shown that the penumbra may persist for more than 12 h.

Today, an increasing number of centers use MRI, including perfusion/diffusion-weighted imaging (PWI/DWI), as a diagnostic tool for hyperacute stroke before deciding on therapy.

*Example*
With the introduction of non-invasive imaging, such as magnetic resonance imaging with the stroke sensitive sequence "DWI," growth of brain infarcts could be shown.

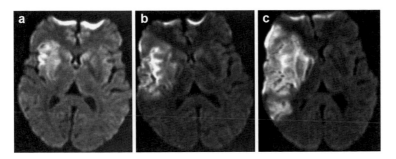

**Fig. 1.6** Magnetic resonance diffusion-weighted imaging (DWI) after 20 minutes (**a**), 3 hours (**b**), and 6 hours (**c**)

In the infarct core, cell injury is established within minutes (Fig. 1.6a). During the following sub-acute phase, the infarct core expands into the peri-infarct penumbra (Fig. 1.6b) until, after 4–6 h, the core spreads into the entire penumbra area (Fig. 1.6c). Subsequently, vasogenic edema and inflammation contribute to further changes such as swelling that can cause further damage and even fatal brain herniation.

Perfusion/diffusion-weighted (PW/DW) – magnetic resonance imaging is the most widely available and most utilized method to detect tissue amenable for therapy in patients with acute stroke, and it is therefore the preferred method for the selection of patients and for the evaluation of treatment effects in stroke trials (Heiss 2010). However, the perfusion-weighted imaging abnormality often overestimates the final infarct volume and thereby the amount of tissue at risk. Also, the initial diffusion lesion does not only consist of irreversibly infarcted tissue. It was shown that, if blood flow is restored at an early time-point, these diffusion lesions can even be reversed (Heiss 2010).

### 1.4.3 Physiologic and Imaging Changes

In ischemic stroke, either by complete or partial occlusion of the supplying vessels, the affected brain tissue can no longer keep up its metabolic requirements, namely, those of nutrient supply and waste disposal. This results in loss of neuronal electrical activity and the depletion of cellular energy stores. Without this energy, the transmembrane ion pumps can no longer keep up the physiological balance between water, sodium, chloride, and potassium. What follows is the redistribution of water from the extracellular to the intracellular space causing swelling of the cells.

1

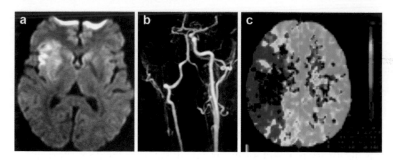

**Fig. 1.7** (**a–c**) MR-PWI/DWI. Diffusion-weighted MRI (DWI) demonstrates a hyper-intense, small infarct in the right middle cerebral artery (MCA) territory (**a**). Contrast enhanced MR-Angiography (CE–MRA) reveals an occlusion of the right carotid artery (**b**). Although at the time of infarct, only a small infarct core is visible, perfusion weighted MRI (**c**) already depicts "tissue at risk" that involves the complete MCA territory. If timely recanalization cannot be achieved, a complete, right-sided MCA infarct will develop

Discrimination between infarct core and surrounding potentially salvageable tissue (penumbra) is important so as to better identify patients suitable for treatment.

This can be achieved by CT perfusion scans or MR-PWI/DWI.

*Example*

The patient in Fig. 1.7 had a sudden onset of left sided hemiparesis that happened 20 min ago. The presumed diagnosis is a stroke in the right brain hemisphere. This is confirmed on magnetic resonance imaging (MRI) using a diffusion-weighted sequence (DWI) that can detect fresh ischemic stroke within minutes of onset (**a**). The underlying cause is an occlusion of the right carotid artery, which is completely missing on the MR-Angiography (**b**). This causes the perfusion deficit (*red area*) in the right hemisphere (**c**) (Fig. 1.7).

Magnetic resonance scanners using diffusion-weighted imaging (DWI) are able to detect the initial ischemic disturbance within minutes after arterial occlusion.

Diffusion-perfusion magnetic resonance imaging (DWI/PWI) is increasingly available at major hospitals worldwide for the acute evaluation of ischemic stroke patients. Despite the fact that in clinical routine, perfusion estimation is not truly quantitative, and PW imaging abnormalities are sometimes overestimated, this technique has been shown a valuable tool for identification of tissue at risk, the tissue that is still amenable to treatment.

The hyper-intense areas on DWI are generally believed to represent the irreversible ischemic changes, but very early changes in diffusion can even be reversed by timely intervention. Perfusion-weighted imaging requires the intravenous administration of contrast media and gives information on the current brain tissue perfusion. The PWI/DWI mismatch region, defined as the difference in volume of tissue between the smaller diffusion lesion and the larger perfusion deficit, is thought to approximately correspond to the ischemic penumbra.

Over the last years, fast scanners have made CT perfusion a reality. With these scans, the cerebral blood flow and cerebral blood volume can be evaluated.

Disadvantages in identifying the penumbra with perfusion CT are:

- It can only cover a limited volume of brain.
- It is necessary to inject a substantial amount of iodinated contrast, which may later add to the amount of contrast needed in neuro-intervention.
- It necessitates the use of radiation.

Whatever method is used, timely discrimination between infarct core and the surrounding potentially salvageable tissue is necessary to better identify patients suitable for acute stroke treatment. As tissue tolerance to ischemic damage depends on the residual flow and the duration of occlusion, ischemic penumbra is a dynamic process. This makes the time window of therapeutic opportunity variable, ill-defined, and highly individual. Obviously, it is shortest for the core of ischemia but may extend to several hours in the under-perfused surrounding penumbral brain tissue where blood flow is sufficiently reduced to cause hypoxia and severe enough to inhibit all physiological function, but not so complete as to cause irreversible cell death.

> Discrimination between infarct core and surrounding potentially salvageable tissue (penumbra) is important so as to better identify patients suitable for treatment. This can be achieved by CT perfusion scans or MR-PWI/DWI.

### 1.4.4   What Are the Treatment Options in Hyper-acute Stroke?

The treatment of ischemic stroke aims to reopen the occluded blood vessel as quickly as possible by dissolving or removing the clot that is preventing brain perfusion.

The most effective stroke treatment can only be administered in the early hours after the onset of stroke.

> Basically, treatment options today for hyper-acute stroke comprise of:
>
> (a) "Lysis," meaning the intravenous or intra-arterial administration of a medication to dissolve the clot.
> (b) Mechanical recanalization using endovascular devices directly in the brain.

### 1.4.5   What Is Lysis?

"*Lysis*" derives from the Greek word λ σις, *lýsis* (from *lýein*) and means "to separate." It refers to the breaking down of the clot formation.

There are various drugs used for thrombolytic therapy. The most commonly used drugs are recombinant tissue plasminogen activator (rtPA) and urokinase.

Both thrombolytic agents are serine proteases that work by converting plasminogen to the natural fibrinolytic agent plasmin. Plasmin then lyses the clot by breaking down the fibrinogen and fibrin it contains. If no fibrin is present, fibrin-specific thrombolytic agents can only convert very little plasminogen to plasmin.

> *Urokinase* (urokinase-type plasminogen activator) got its name as it was originally isolated from urine. It directly activates plasminogen to form plasmin.
>
> When purified from human urine, 1,500 l of urine are needed to gain enough urokinase to treat a single patient. It is also commercially available in a form produced by tissue culture. Recombinant DNA techniques have been developed for urokinase production in *E. coli* cultures.
>
> *Tissue plasminogen activator (tPA)* is a physiologically occurring fibrinolytic that can be found in the endothelial cells of the vessels. It regulates the balance between thrombolysis and thrombus formation agents and degrades fibrin clots through activation of plasminogen to plasmin. In the absence of fibrin, fibrin-specific thrombolytic agents (alteplase (rtPA), tenecteplase, and reteplase) induce only plasmin, whereas non–fibrin-specific agents such as streptokinase will catalyze systemic fibrinolysis. Streptokinase is thus not indicated in acute ischemic stroke but continues to be used because of its lower cost.

Alteplase (rtPA) is currently the only lytic agent approved by the FDA (US Food and Drug Administration) for acute ischemic stroke. It has been shown efficient in reducing disability after ischemic stroke.

However, new agents are under investigation, and the choice of lytic agents will be based upon the results of further clinical trials.

Lysis can be given intravenously or intra-arterially, directly into the clot. For intra-arterial lysis, a special, small catheter (micro-catheter) is inserted via the femoral artery of the leg and is then placed into the occluded intracranial vessel (Fig. 1.8). Ideally, the catheter is passed adjacent to the thrombus where the injection of lytics can be locally, rather than systemically, delivered.

However, as in intravenous lysis, delayed treatment with late administration of tissue-type plasminogen activator (tPA) is associated with an increasingly higher risk of cerebral bleed or hemorrhagic transformation, the major complications of antithrombotic and thrombolytic therapy that can result in further brain damage.

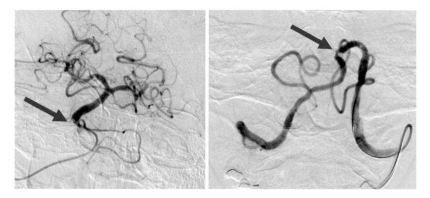

**Fig. 1.8** A micro-catheter is placed into the left vertebral artery, and intra-arterial lysis is administered directly in front of the occluded basilar artery

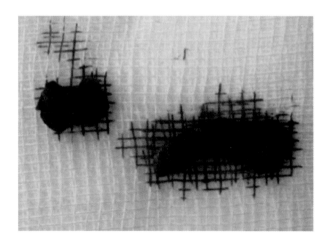

**Fig. 1.9** Image of an intracranial thrombus that was aspirated using the Penumbra$^{TR}$ device

## 1.5 Pathophysiology of Thrombosis

### 1.5.1 How Does Lysis Work?

When a vascular insult occurs, immediate local cellular response takes place. Platelets migrate to the area of injury where they secrete several cellular factors and mediators. These mediators promote the clot formation (Fig. 1.9).

Intra-venous fibrinolysis is, to date, the most commonly used intervention in acute stroke.

However, over the last years, endovascular interventions have shown very promising results with intra-arterial administration of thrombolytics as well as mechanical clot retrieving methods.

The normal hemostatic response that limits bleeding is thrombosis. This physiologic thrombosis is counterbalanced by intrinsic antithrombotic

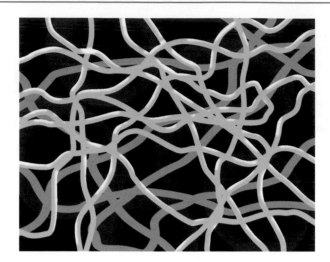

**Fig. 1.10** Thrombus formation: circulating prothrombin is activated to thrombin (active clotting factor) by activated platelets. This newly activated thrombin activates fibrinogen to fibrin. Fibrin is then formed into a fibrin mesh. At the same time, platelets are aggregated and plasminogen gathers in the fibrin matrix

mechanisms and fibrinolysis. Normally, a thrombus is confined to the immediate area of injury and would not obstruct blood flow.

In a stroke, however, the thrombus has occluded an artery, thus impairing the normal hemodynamic function.

During thrombus formation, circulating prothrombin is activated to thrombin. This newly activated thrombin activates fibrinogen to fibrin. Fibrin is then formed into a fibrin mesh. At the same time, platelets are aggregated (Fig. 1.10).

Thus, the three main components of a blood clot are:

• Platelets
• Thrombin
• Fibrin

Antiplatelet drugs such as aspirin, glycoprotein IIb/IIIa inhibitors, and clopidogrel have an inhibitory effect on platelet aggregation, but all have failed to prove effective for recanalization of acutely obstructed cerebral vessels.

Thrombolytic drugs such as rtPA and urokinase degrade the fibrin clot through activation of the enzyme plasminogen, which directly attacks the fibrin mesh.

They can therefore actively reduce the size of the clot, while other anticoagulants (such as heparin) will mainly decrease the "growth."

However, the thrombolysis process works best on recently formed thrombus as older thrombi have an extensive fibrin polymerization that makes them very resistant to thrombolysis (Fig. 1.11).

**Fig. 1.11**
Thrombolytic drugs
degrade the fibrin
clot through
activation of the
enzyme
plasminogen, which
directly attacks the
fibrin mesh

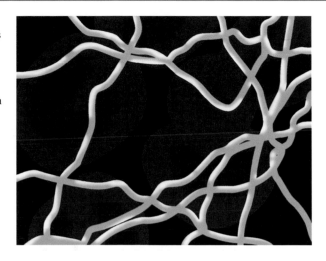

## 1.6   Understanding That "Time Is Brain"

Although irreversible cell death begins within minutes after stroke onset
within the core of the infarct, not all brain cells will die simultaneously.
This is because our brain is supplied with blood from four distinct and
interconnecting vessels. Most of the tissues of the brain can get some
blood from collateral circulation despite the occlusion of the primary
source. Thus, for several hours, there exists a surrounding volume of tissue
that is at risk for infarction but yet potentially salvageable (tissue at risk).
With every minute, the extent of viable tissue diminishes, and any
recanalization attempt will be less and less effective.

The average number of neurons in the human forebrain is 22 billion.
The average duration of large vessel stroke evolution is 10 hours and
ranges between 6 and 18 hours.

In 1 hour of a typical large vessel ischemic stroke a patient loses:
- 120 million neurons
- 830 billion synapses
- 714 km of myelinated fibers
  In each minute a patient loses:
- 3.9 million neurons
- 1.4 billion synapses
- 12 km of myelinated fibers (Saver 2006)

**Fig. 1.12** The stroke chain for integrated care

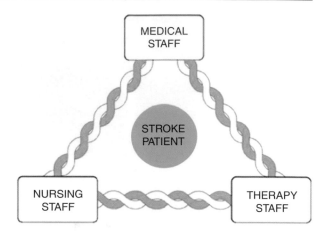

## 1.7    What Is a Stroke Pathway?

With stroke ranked as one of the most costly diseases for the elderly, acute and hyper-acute stroke services and pathways are increasingly initiated to improve the management and outcome of stroke patients. A coherent stroke pathway can be defined as the organization of a chain of caregivers, including medical, nursing, and therapy staff, who, together as a team, enable expert and integrated care for stroke patients through all phases – i.e., hyper-acute, acute, rehabilitation, and chronic.

This will necessitate regional co-operation between the disciplines and institutions involved.

Though there are different ways to organize an acute stroke service, some common elements are a predefined emergency chain that includes imaging, a specialist multidisciplinary medical team, a stroke unit, and agreements about transfers from one hospital or institution to another, for further specialist clinical management or rehabilitation to minimize discharge delays.

## 1.8    Where Should Stroke Care Take Place?

Stroke care should take place in a dedicated stroke unit that facilitates the integration of specialized medical, nursing, and therapy staff (Fig. 1.12).

General stroke care includes prevention of hypoxia, blood pressure and glucose control, maintenance of euthermia, and nutritional support.

In 2002, an analysis by the Stroke Unit Trialists showed an 18% relative reduction in mortality, reduction in death or dependence, and a reduction in death or need of institutional care when patients were treated in a stroke unit, as compared to being treated in a general medical ward (level I evidence). The absolute changes indicated a 3% reduction in all cause

**Fig. 1.13** The different disciplines in a stroke unit

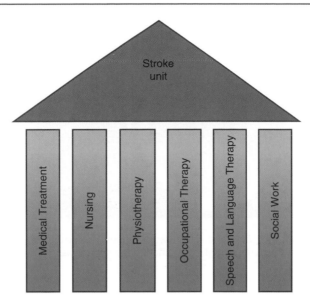

mortality (number needed to treat (NNT) 33), a 3% reduction in the need for nursing home care, and a 6% increase in the number of independent survivors (NNT 16).

All types of patients, regardless of gender, age, and severity of stroke profited from treatment in stroke units (Stroke Unit Trialists' Collaboration 2002).

## 1.9   What Is a Stroke Unit?

A stroke unit is a unit within the hospital that exclusively or nearly exclusively takes care of stroke patients. It provides a coordinated, multidisciplinary approach to treatment and care. The different disciplines in such a team are medical treatment, nursing, physiotherapy, occupational therapy, speech and language therapy, and social work (Fig. 1.13). It should have the facilities of a neurological intensive care unit, headed by a neuro-intensivist with appropriate training to handle all stroke patients.

## 1.10   What Is Decompressive Craniectomy?

Neurosurgical decompressive craniectomy in large ischemic stroke is, by now, a well-described and accepted procedure in which a section of the skull is removed to allow swelling brain room to expand. This relieves intracranial pressure and gives the brain a place to swell without inducing more damage.

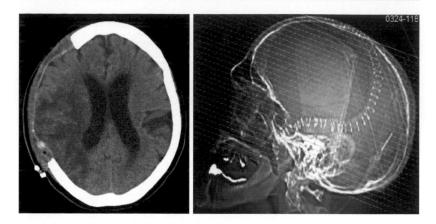

**Fig. 1.14**  *Left*: decompressive craniectomy was performed to allow parenchymal swelling after a right-sided MCA infarct. *Right*: replacement of the skull fragment

Usually, only younger patients (below 60 years) are treated, based on the first study populations and the fact that these patients are of higher risk for intracranial brain pressure due to the absence of brain atrophy.

Until today, five randomized controlled trials on decompressive surgery in stroke patients have been conducted: two North American and three European studies (Vahedi et al. 2007a, b; Juttler et al. 2007; Hofmeijer et al. 2009; Frank 2010; Jamora 2010).

The evidence, especially in younger patients, is that they are more likely to survive when undergoing decompressive craniectomy early (within 48 h of stroke onset). However, the increased survival rate is at the cost of a higher likelihood of moderate to moderately severe disability (Schirmer et al. 2008) (Fig. 1.14).

## 1.11   What Is Neuroprotection in Stroke?

There have been several attempts to save ischemic neurons in the penumbra from irreversible damage using neuroprotective drugs. This is a promising area of pharmaceutical research. Examples are the modulation of neuronal receptors so that excitatory neurotransmitters, which contribute to early neuronal injury, are not released. Although promising results have already been achieved in animal experimental work, transfer of such treatments to the human stroke patient has not been achieved so far.

The therapeutic benefits of hypothermia in patients with acute ischemic stroke are currently under research. Hypothermia appears to be a promising neuroprotective therapy, as it affects a wide range of destructive mechanisms occurring in ischemic brain tissue. Animal research has substantiated its use in acute ischemic stroke. The European Hypothermia Stroke Research Workshop, organized by the European Stroke Research Network for Hypothermia (EuroHyp), was held in January 2010. An imminent aim is to validate therapeutic cooling as a novel treatment. A proposed integrated Phase II and III clinical study program shall test the effectiveness of this intervention and would allow the development of evidence-based Clinical Practice Guidelines for hypothermia as a treatment strategy for stroke (Macleod et al. 2010).

## References

Bernard CDC, Iburg KM, Inoue M, Ma Fat D, Shibuya K, Stein C, Tomijima T, Xu H (2003) Global burden of disease in 2002: data sources, methods and results. http://www.who.int/infobase. Accessed 20 Apr 2011

Bogousslavsky J, Paciaroni M (2009) The economics of treating stroke as an acute brain attack. BMC Med 7:51

Branston NM, Hope DT, Symon L (1979) Barbiturates in focal ischemia of primate cortex: effects on blood flow distribution, evoked potential and extracellular potassium. Stroke 10:647–653

Cadilhac D, Dewey H et al. (2005) Investing in stroke – what are the potential cost offsets from the strokesafe program. National Stroke Research Institute – Technical Report (unpublished)

Caro JJ, Huybrechts KF (1999) Stroke treatment economic model (STEM): predicting long term costs from functional status. Stroke 30:2574–2579

Caro JJ et al (2000) Management of patterns and costs of acute ischemic stroke; an international study. Stroke 31:582–590

Evers SMAA, Struijs JN, Ament AJHA, van Genugten MLL, Jager JC, van den Bos GAM (2002) The disease impact, health care management, and costs of stroke in the Netherlands. Report 282701001/2002, National Institute for Public Health and the Environment (RIVM), Bilthoven

Frank JI. Hemicraniectomy and durotomy for deterioration from infarction relating swelling trial (HeaDDFIRST). Stroke trials registry. http://www.strokecenter.org/trials/trialDetail.aspx?tid=70&search_string=headdfirst. Accessed 23 Aug 2010.

Heart and Stroke Foundation of Canada (2003) The growing burden of heart disease and stroke in Canada 2003. The Foundation, Ottawa. www.cvdinfobase.ca/cvdbook/CVD_En03.pdf. Accessed 19 Apr 2011

Heiss WD (2010) The concept of the penumbra: can it be translated to stroke management? Int J Stroke 5(4):290–295

Hofmeijer J, Kappelle LJ, Algra A et al (2009) Surgical decompression for space-occupying cerebral infarction (the hemicraniectomy after middle cerebral artery infarction with life-threatening edema trial [HAMLET]): a multicentre, open, randomised trial. Lancet Neurol 8:326–333

Huijsman R, Klazinga NS, Scholte op Reimer WJM, van Wijngaarden JDH, van Exel NJA, van Putte-Boon C, Prestholt FT, Koopmanschap MA, Niessen LW (2001) Beroerte, beroering en borging in de keten: results of the EDISSE study of three regional experiments with stroke-service [in Dutch]. Report, ZonMW, the Hague

Isard PA, Forbes JF (1992) The cost of stroke to the National Health Service in Scotland. Cerebrovasc Dis 5:47–50

Jamora RD. Hemicraniectomy for malignant middle cerebral artery infarcts (HeMMI).
    Stroke trials registry. http://www.strokecenter.org/trials/trialDetail.aspx?tid=575.
    Accessed 23 Aug 2010
Juttler E, Schwab S, Schmiedek P (2007) Decompressive surgery for the treatment of
    malignant infarction of the middle cerebral artery (DESTINY): a randomized, con-
    trolled trial. Stroke 38:2518–2525
Kleindorfer DLC, White G, Curtis T, Brass L, Koroshetz W, Broderick JP (2008) National
    US estimates of rt-PA use: ICD-9 codes substantially underestimate. Stroke 39:924–928
Macleod MR, Petersson J, Norrving B, Hacke W, Dirnagl U, Wagner M, Schwab S,
    European Hypothermia Stroke Research Workshop (2010) Hypothermia for stroke:
    call to action 2010. Int J Stroke 5(6):489–492
Mant J, Wade DT, Winner S (2004) Health care needs assessment: stroke. In: Stevens A, Raftery
    J, Mant J et al (eds) Health care needs assessment: the epidemiologically based needs
    assessment reviews, 2nd edn, First series. Radcliffe Medical Press, Oxford, pp 141–244
Nagahiro S, Uno M, Sato K, Goto S, Morioka M, Ushio Y (1998) Pathophysiology and
    treatment of cerebral ischemia. J Med Invest 45:57–70
National Sentinel Stroke Audit Phase II (clinical audit) (2008) Clinical effectiveness and
    evaluation unit. Report for England, Wales and Northern Ireland. Royal College of
    Physicians of London, London
Reddy K, Yusuf S (1998) Emerging epidemic of cardiovascular disease in developing
    countries. Circulation 97:596–601
Reinhardt E (2005) The Atlas of heart disease and stroke. (HealthWatch): An article
    from: UN Chronicle (p. 8). United Nations Publications
Saver JL (2006) Time is brain—quantified. Stroke 37:263–266
Schirmer CM, Ackil AA Jr, Malek AM (2008) Decompressive craniectomy. Neurocrit
    Care 8:456–470
Stroke Unit Trialists' Collaboration (2002) Organised inpatient (stroke unit) care for
    stroke. Cochrane Database Syst Rev 1:CD000197, Update in: Cochrane Database
    Syst Rev 2007;(4):CD000197
Study Cohort 1991.
The Erlangen stroke project (2006) Lifetime cost of ischemic stroke in Germany: results
    and national projections from a population based stroke registry. Stroke 37:1179–1183
Vahedi K, Vicaut E, Mateo J et al (2007a) Sequential design, multi-center, randomized,
    controlled trial of early decompressive craniectomy in malignant middle cerebral
    artery infarction (DECIMAL trial). Stroke 38:2506–2517
Vahedi K, Hofmeijer J, Juettler E et al (2007b) Early decompressive surgery in malignant
    infarction of the middle cerebral artery: a pooled analysis of three randomized ran-
    domized trials. Lancet Neurol 6(3):215–222
Warlow CP, Dennis MS, van Gijn J, Sandercock PAG, Bamford JM, Wardlaw JM (2001)
    Stroke: a practical guide to management. Blackwell Science, Oxford
Wolf PA, D'Agostino RB, Belanger AJ, Kannel WB (1991) Probability of stroke: a risk
    profile from the Framingham Study. Stroke 22(3):312–318

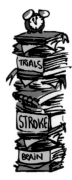

## Further Reading

Back T (1998) Pathophysiology of the ischemic penumbra–revision of a concept. Cell
    Mol Neurobiol 18(6):621–638, Review
Merenda A, DeGeorgia M (2010) Craniectomy for acute stroke: how to apply the data to
    the bedside. Curr Opin Neurol 23:53

# Guidelines and Regulations

**2**

## 2.1    Sources of Supporting Information

Evidence-based guidelines are an important contribution to efficient and cost-effective management of acute stroke. Such guidelines aim at providing recommendations for high quality and equal level of care to the national and international medical community and represent a common basis for the optimal management of acute stroke. The adherence to these guidelines may or may not play an important role in the outcome of acute stroke patients.

Guidelines and recommendations are certainly a valuable tool for clinicians involved in the treatment of acute stroke patients. A considerable number of guidelines covering different aspects of acute stroke management have been published over the last decade. However, too many guidelines with different and sometimes conflicting recommendations may make it difficult for some clinicians to decide which guidelines to follow. Detailed guidelines are helpful – but they have to be updated regularly to keep pace with the fast development in acute stroke treatment.

The American Heart Association/American Stroke Association has issued one of the best-known guidelines. The AHA ASA has published separate guidelines on management of acute ischemic stroke, which were published in 1994. As new scientific evidence becomes available based on controlled stroke trials, many guidelines have and will continue to be updated. For example, the AHA ASA guidelines of 1994 were amended soon after in 1996, when the US Food and Drug Administration (FDA) had approved thrombolytic therapy in ischemic stroke. They were again amended in 2009, when the time window for treatment of acute ischemic stroke with intravenous tissue plasminogen activator was expanded to 4.5 h – based on the results of the ECASS-III study (although labeling for the drug has not yet been adapted for use beyond the 3 h time window).

I.Q. Grunwald et al., *How to set up an Acute Stroke Service*,
DOI 10.1007/978-3-642-21405-9_2, © Springer-Verlag Berlin Heidelberg 2012

Besides the AHA ASA, other main American guidelines are those published by the National Institute of Neurological Disorders and Stroke (NINDS) and the National Stroke Association (NSA) which also include guidelines on stroke *prevention*, namely the guidelines for the prevention of stroke in patients with stroke or transient ischemic attack published in 2010 by the AHA ASA. The aim of this new statement is to provide comprehensive and timely evidence-based recommendations on the prevention of ischemic stroke among survivors of previous ischemic stroke or transient ischemic attack.

European clinicians may find it useful to apply the American guidelines or choose between a multitude of local, national, and international guidelines. For example, due to discrepancies between the different local health care resources, some local or national guidelines and recommendations cannot be applied at a specific hospital, e.g., lack of CT or MRI facilities, laboratory availability, or 24-h monitoring.

Finland was one of the first countries to publish national guidelines. Some national guidelines may represent a reliable source of evidence-based information on different aspects of acute stroke management, but a more homogenous presentation should facilitate the clinicians' task. Also, some recommendations, such as the WHO consensus statement, are too general to be efficiently implemented in the daily clinical decision-making.

International organizations have also issued guidelines, such as the European Federation of Neurological Societies (EFNS), which published its guidelines for acute stroke care in 1997.

More recently, the European Stroke Organization (ESO) published guidelines for management of ischemic stroke in 2008, which have been updated in 2009 with regard to thrombolytic therapy. These guidelines represent an update of the European Stroke Initiative (EUSI) guidelines published in 2000 and cover referral and emergency management, stroke unit service, diagnostics, primary and secondary prevention, general stroke treatment, specific treatment including acute management, management of complications, and rehabilitation.

The last decade was characterized by the implementation of stroke units for acute stroke patients together with a number of relevant national guidelines and recommendations. The recommendations for the establishment of primary stroke centers by the Brain Attack Coalition (BAC) published in 2000 address eleven major aspects of acute stroke care.

Furthermore, the ESO guidelines give a comprehensive overview of the organization of prehospital and in-hospital pathways and systems for acute stroke patients and recommend that acute stroke patients should be treated in stroke units.

Randomized clinical trials have shown that stroke units tend to increase survival rates among acute stroke patients as compared to general medical wards. Many different approaches to stroke unit organizations exist, e.g.:

• Acute stroke units focusing on skilled treatment for patients in the acute phase
• Nonintensive stroke units or stroke rehabilitation units
• Comprehensive stroke units combining acute and rehabilitation stroke care

Some of these are in the process of being certified according to criteria for optimal care of acute stroke patients.

Another international recommendation is the creation of mobile stroke teams in both acute care and rehabilitation hospitals. The aim here is to provide skilled treatment at every stage of the disease to those hospitals without own resources.

Over the last decade, telemedicine using a bidirectional videoconferencing equipment to provide health services or assist health care personnel in remote rural areas are emerging. They are seen as a potential timesaving and efficient means for evaluating patients experiencing acute stroke. Telemedicine may link an emergency department physician with a distant specialist in a stroke unit. Relevant statements are included, among others, in the recommendations for the implementation of telemedicine within stroke systems of care published in 2009 by the AHA ASA as well as in the ESO guidelines, but many questions remain unresolved, i.e., legal issues when giving indication for high-risk treatments of remote patients without adequate personal investigation.

Due to the increasing number of local, national, and international recommendations and guidelines, there seems to be an obvious need for critical evaluation and harmonization of available guidelines. Yet, although current guidelines differ in their variety, taking into account cultural and economic factors, they represent a solid instrument to assist the clinicians in daily acute stroke care.

As indicated by the ESO, global harmonization of stroke guidelines will be the focus of the World Stroke Organization, supported by the ESO and other national and regional stroke societies.

## 2.2    Guidelines

The following tables include an extract of the list of currently existing stroke guidelines identified through members of the World Stroke Organization (Tables 2.1–2.7).

**Table 2.1** Stroke care across the continuum (prehospital, acute care, rehabilitation, and prevention)

| Guideline | Organization | Country | Year |
|---|---|---|---|
| Canadian best practice recommendations for stroke care (2008 update). Available: CMAJ 2008; 179: E1–E93 | Canadian stroke strategy | Canada | 2008 |
| Chilean stroke guidelines | Cerebrovascular Diseases Group | Chile | 2008 |
| Stroke guideline | Chinese Neurological Society | China | 2007 |
| Guideline of cerebrovascular diseases treatment | Institute of Medicine in Shanghai | China | 2008–2011 |
| Guideline for stroke management | Chinese Stroke Association | China | 2008 |
| China guideline for cerebrovascular disease prevention and treatment | Neurology Commission Branch of CMA | China | 2008 |
| Demarin V, Lovren I, Huzjan A, et al. Recommendations for stroke management (2006 update). Available: Acta Clin Croat 2006; 45:219–285 | Croatian Society for Neurovascular Disorders | Croatia | 2006 |
| Guidelines for management of ischemic stroke and transient ischemic attack | European Stroke Organization | Europe | 2008 |
| Aivoinfarkti (stroke) | Task Force nominated by the Finnish Neurological Association together with the Finnish Medical Society Duodecim | Finland | 2006 |
| Kaypa hoito (current care) | National Stroke Group | Finland | 2006 |
| Guidelines stroke 2007 | Pokja Stroke Perdossi (Stroke Task Force Indonesian Neurological Association) | Yogyakarta Indonesia | 2007 |
| Spread stroke prevention Italian guidelines | SPREAD Italy | Italy | 2007 |
| Nacionaini vodi za lije enjeakutnog mo danog udara | Neurological Society of Serbia & Montenegro | Montenegro | 2004 |
| Life after stroke: New Zealand guideline for management of stroke | Stroke Foundation of New Zealand | New Zealand | 2003 |
| New Zealand TIA guideline | New Zealand Guideline Group | New Zealand | 2008 |
| Guidelines for stroke management | Stroke Society of the Philippines | Philippines | 2006 |
| Guideline about stroke and TIA management in 2008 | Romanian Association of Stroke | Romania | 2008 |

| Nationella riktlinjer for strokevard | National Board of Health & Welfare | Sweden | 2005 |
|---|---|---|---|
| National stroke guidelines | National Board of Health & Welfare | Sweden | 2006 |
| Inselspital, University of Bern (H. Mattle) | ZAS | Switzerland | 2007 |
| Guidelines for stroke prevention | Neurological Society of Thailand | Thailand | 2007 |
| National stroke guidelines 3rd edition | Royal College of Physicians | United Kingdom | 2008 |
| Stroke guidelines | National Institute for Health and Clinical Excellence (NICE) | United Kingdom | 2008 |
| SIGN 64: management of patients with stroke: rehabilitation, prevention, and management of complications, and discharge planning | Scottish Intercollegiate Guidelines Network (SIGN) | United Kingdom | 2006 |

**Table 2.2** Prehospital (emergency medical services) stroke care

| | | | |
|---|---|---|---|
| (doi: 10.1590/S0004282X2002000400032) | Academia Brasileira de Neurologica | Brazil | 2002 |
| The recognition and emergency management of suspected stroke and TIA guidelines supplement | Royal College of Physicians (RCP) National Pre-Hospital Guidelines Group | United Kingdom | 2006 |
| Guideline for the management of acute ischemic stroke | American Heart Association | United States | 2007 |
| Guidelines for the management of spontaneous hemorrhage in adults | American Heart Association | United States | 2007 |
| Guidelines for the Management of transient ischemic attack | American Heart Association | United States | 1994 |

**Table 2.3** Acute and rehabilitation components

| | | | |
|---|---|---|---|
| Clinical guidelines for stroke rehabilitation and recovery | National stroke foundation | Australia | 2005 |
| Best practice guideline for stroke care | Heart & Stroke Foundation of Canada | Canada | 2003 |
| Nursing best practice guideline: stroke assessment across the continuum of care | Registered Nurses Association of Ontario (RNAO) | Canada | 2005 |
| Nova Scotia guidelines for stroke care | Cardiovascular Health Nova Scotia | Canada | 2008 |
| Japanese guidelines for the management of stroke available: Int J Stroke; 2008: 3: 55–62 | The Joint Committee (Japan Stroke Society, and other four stroke-related Japanese societies) | Japan | 2004 |
| Up-to-date principles of diagnostics and management of patients with acute disorders of cerebral perfusion | Ukrainian Anti-Stroke Association | Ukraine | 2007 |

**Table 2.4** Acute stroke care

| | | | |
|---|---|---|---|
| Clinical guidelines for acute stroke management | National stroke foundation | Australia | 2007 |
| Guias de Practica Clinica para la prevencion del accidente cerebrovascular isquemico y el ataque isquemico transitorio Available: Revista Neurologica Argentina 2006; 31: 74–9 | Sociedad Neurologica Argentina | Argentina | 2006 |
| Primeiro Consenso Brasileira | Sociedade Brasileira de Doencas Cerebrovasculares | Brazil | |

**Table 2.4**  (continued)

| Clinical practice guidelines for hemorrhagic stroke | Neurological Society of Thailand | Thailand | 2004 |
|---|---|---|---|
| Guideline stroke | Pokja Stroke Perdossi (Stroke Task Force Indonesian Neurological Association) | Indonesia | 2008 |
| SIGN 108 management of patients with stroke or TIA | Scottish Intercollegiate Guidelines Network (SIGN) | United Kingdom | 2008 |
| Stroke assessment: booklet for patients | Scottish Intercollegiate Guidelines Network (SIGN) | United Kingdom | 2008 |
| SIGN 78:management of patients with stroke: identification and management of dysphagia | Scottish Intercollegiate Guidelines Network (SIGN) | United Kingdom | 2004 |
| Stroke in childhood: clinical guidelines for diagnosis, management and rehabilitation | Royal College of Physicians (RCP) Pediatric Stroke Working Group | United Kingdom | 2004 |
| Stroke guidelines | Society Against Stroke in Ukraine (SASU) | Ukraine | 2007 |
| Guidelines for the early management of adults with ischemic stroke. Available: Stroke 2007; 38: 1655–1711 | American Heart Association | United States | 2007 |
| Guidelines for the management of spontaneous intracerebral hemorrhage in adults: 2007 update Available: Stroke 2007; 38: 2001–2023 | American Heart Association | United States | 2007 |
| Management of stroke in infants and children: a scientific statement for healthcare professionals from a special writing group of the stroke council. Available: Stroke 2008; 39: 2644–91 | American Heart Association | United States | 2008 |

**Table 2.5**  Stroke rehabilitation

| Clinical guidelines for stroke rehabilitation and recovery http://www.strokefoundation.com.au/post-acute-health-professional | National stroke foundation | Australia | 2005 |
|---|---|---|---|
| Stroke care optimization of rehabilitation through evidence (SCORE) | SCORE Research Group | Canada | 2007 |
| Ottawa panel evidence-based clinical practice guidelines for post-stroke rehabilitation Available: Top Stroke Rehabil 2006; 13(2): 1–269 | Ottawa Panel Research Group | Canada | 2006 |
| EBRSR: evidence-based review of stroke rehabilitation. 11th ed. London (ON): EBRSR; 2008 | EBRSR Research Group | Canada | 2008 |

(continued)

**Table 2.5**   (continued)

| Clinical practice guidelines for hemorrhagic stroke | Neurological Society of Thailand | Thailand | 2004 |
|---|---|---|---|
| Management of adult stroke rehabilitation care: a clinical practice guideline. Available: Stroke 2005; 36: e100–e143 | American Heart Association | Unites States | 2005 |
| Clinical practice guidelines for the management of stroke rehabilitation | Veterans Affairs/ Department of Defense | United States | 2003 |

**Table 2.6**   Stroke prevention (secondary)

| Neuroprotective agents in stroke: nacional opinión. Arq Neuropsiquiatr 2005; 63: 889–91 | Doencas cerebrovasculares | Brazil | 2005 |
|---|---|---|---|
| Management of carotid disease in acute phase of stroke: nacional opinión. Arq Neuropsiquiatr 2005; 63(3A): 709–12 | Sociedade Brasileira de Doencas Cerebrovasculares | Brazil | 2005 |
| Guidelines for the prevention of stroke in patients with ischemic stroke or TIA. Available: Stroke 2006; 37: 577–617 | American Heart Association | United States | 2006 |

**Table 2.7**   Stroke prevention (primary)

| Primary prevention of ischemic stroke. A guideline from the American Heart Association/American Stroke Association Stroke Council. Stroke 2006; 37: 1583–1633 | American Heart Association | United States | 2006 |
|---|---|---|---|

Source: http://www.world-stroke.org/guidelines_hb02.asp last access April 2011

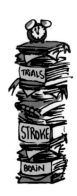

# Further Reading

Adams HP Jr, del Zoppo G, Alberts MJ, Bhatt DL, Brass L et al (2007) Guidelines for the early management of adults with ischemic stroke: a guideline from the American Heart Association/American Stroke Association Stroke Council, Clinical Cardiology Council, Cardiovascular Radiology and Intervention Council, and the Atherosclerotic Peripheral Vascular Disease and Quality of Care Outcomes in Research Interdisciplinary Working Groups: The American Academy of Neurology affirms the value of this guideline as an educational tool for neurologists. Circulation 115:e478–e534

European Stroke Organization (ESO) Executive Committee: Collective Name: ESO Writing Committee (2008) Guidelines for management of ischemic stroke and transient ischemic attack. Cerebrovasc Dis 25:457–507

http://www.americanheart.org. Last accessed May 2011

http://www.ninds.nih.gov. Last accessed May 2011

http://www.stroke.org. Last accessed May 2011

http://www.efns.org. Last accessed May 2011

http://www.eso-stroke.org. Last accessed May 2011

http://www.stroke-site.org. Last accessed May 2011

# Who Can Support This Project?

**3**

## 3.1 Expertise

Setting up a stroke service requires a multidisciplinary approach and support from every member of the future stroke team, including doctors, nurses, stroke coordinators, and emergency and rehabilitation providers.

Often, enthusiasm and the willingness to support this project are more important than previous expertise and medical background.

If you are not familiar with the different aspects of stroke, in addition to reading this book, you should seek advice from an external specialist who will assess your current infrastructure and resources to best comply with your budgetary constraints. Alongside key clinical staff, you will need to involve business managers, a project manager (if not yourself) and other regulatory authorities as well as expertise within the clinical setting.

This needs to be established in the first phase of the project and can later ensure "buy in" by all essential partners.

Part II of this book will give you the tools, technique, and knowledge to handle this challenging task. It will help you understand what is needed for an acute stroke pathway and will also help you choose the right people to involve.

## 3.2 Funding

Adequate reimbursement of modern stroke treatment is an important factor. Utilizing lytics, as well as endovascular devices, generates costs, not only during the acute treatment but also because of increased personnel and continued follow-up for the survivors. Also, hospitals must create and maintain the necessary infrastructure to ensure safe as well as effective acute stroke treatments.

I.Q. Grunwald et al., *How to set up an Acute Stroke Service*,
DOI 10.1007/978-3-642-21405-9_3, © Springer-Verlag Berlin Heidelberg 2012

Reimbursement must therefore reflect the increased costs associated with evolving thrombolytic and interventional therapy, as well as the cost involved in the setup and funding of an acute service.

In different countries, there are different reimbursement mechanisms but also some research pathways that can help with funding the setup and running of a stroke service.

In **Germany**, reimbursement for an acute stroke patient will be secured by the G-DRG system (German Diagnosis Related Groups). If a new technique or device, e.g., endovascular thrombectomy, is not incorporated into an existing DRG, the hospital will not automatically receive payment. However, in this case, there is a temporary reimbursement system that allows hospitals to use new techniques before they are finally coded and reimbursed by DRGs and incorporated into the healthcare system. If an innovative diagnosis or treatment method does not have a DRG code yet, hospitals can submit requests for reimbursement (Hospital Remuneration Law (KHEntgG)), which is then called NUB reimbursement. Comparable reimbursement mechanisms exist in the UK and in some regions of Italy.

In the DRG coding system, several parameters like the main diagnosis and any additional diagnoses are linked to each other. These diagnoses are coded by the so-called ICD-10 codes. The performed procedure itself (e.g., lysis) is coded using so-called OPS codes in combination with additional characteristics such as the patient's comorbidities and age, which are then combined as one DRG code. Each code can thus be assigned a reimbursable price tag.

The InEK (Institut für das Entgeltsystem im Krankenhaus) is the German Agency for the Hospital Payment System. By accumulating data from reporting hospitals, the InEK enables the DRG system to be a "learning system" that can evolve.

In other countries this may be different. In the UK, funding for a stroke service can be secured through different channels, although many imaging and interventional treatments are not yet properly reimbursed. However, regarding stroke, the UK is currently undergoing a change in policy that encourages the setup of acute stroke services. The Department of Health's *NHS Stroke Improvement Programme*, established in December 2007, is focusing on the development of stroke care networks. One important aspect is the unbundling of the stroke tariff. The NHS White Paper, Equity and Excellence: Liberating the NHS, published in July 2010, sets out the Government's plans, where, in the future, the NHS Commissioning Board will be responsible for the structure of the tariff and a monitor will set prices.

Payment by Results (PbR) is the hospital payment system in **England** in which commissioners pay providers a national tariff or price for the number and complexity of patients treated or seen. Following a Consensus Workshop held in February 2011, the Payment by Results Guidance for 2011–12 includes a commitment to support development of stroke care pathways that best meet the needs of each patient. In any case, making a business case can further financial support.

Despite the fact that only a small amount of patients to date receive any acute stroke treatment, health economic analyses have clearly shown significant savings in terms of quality adjusted life years gained.

**In the USA**, Concentric Medical, Inc., provided a general update of the Centers for Medicare and Medicaid Services (CMS) Inpatient Prospective Payment System (IPPS) rule for Fiscal Year (FY) 2011 and relevant information for ischemic stroke intervention.

This paper, entitled "Hospital Inpatient 2011 Medicare Payment and Policy Update", also provides coding and payment information for endovascular mechanical thrombectomy/embolectomy for acute ischemic stroke. It is intended for educational purposes only:

"The Centers for Medicare and Medicaid Services (CMS) final inpatient rule included a market basket update of 2.6% but reduced this amount by 0.25% as required by the Affordable Care Act and applied a −2.9% 'documentation and coding' adjustment linked to the adoption of the Medicare Severity (MS) Diagnosis Related Group (DRG) system. This resulted in an overall adjustment to hospital payments of negative 0.4% or an expected reduction of $440 million dollars compared to FY 2010."

"Hospitals submit inpatient claims to Medicare, Medicaid, and private insurers on the UB-04 billing form (also called the CMS-1450). The UB-04 displays ICD-9-CM diagnosis codes (principal diagnosis and up to 18 additional diagnoses) and ICD-9-CM procedure codes (principal procedure and up to five additional procedure codes) as well as other patient and billing information to describe the patient's stay and use of resources. Many insurers, including Medicare, use a 24-h length of stay to define inpatient hospital care.

Medicare uses a prospective payment system called Diagnosis Related Groups (DRGs) to reimburse hospitals for inpatient stays. Each inpatient stay is assigned a DRG that is determined according to the principal diagnosis, major procedures, discharge status, and complicating secondary diagnoses. Each DRG is assigned a flat payment rate, which is adjusted according to the individual hospital's teaching status, disproportionate share services for treating low-income patients, and location in urban versus rural regions. DRGs do not include payment for physician services, which are coded and reimbursed separately."

"Other health insurers may reimburse hospitals for inpatient care using per diem rates, DRGs, case rates, or a percentage of charges. Some health insurers may also provide separate payment for single-use disposable devices, such as the Merci Retrieval System™, used in endovascular mechanical embolectomy/thrombectomy procedures."

"International Classification of Diseases (ICD)-9-CM Procedure Code:

By definition, code 39.74 is assigned for procedures using mechanical methods of removing embolus or thrombus, including the Merci Retrieval

**Table 3.1** MS-DRG 23 and 24

| 2011 MS-DRG | Description | Relative weight | 2011 National Average Urban Payment | Average length of stay |
|---|---|---|---|---|
| 23 | Craniotomy w major device implant or acute complex CNS PDX w MCC | 5.0883 | $28,414 | 11.8 |
| 24 | Craniotomy w major device implant or acute complex CNS PDX w/o MCC | 3.4952 | $19,518 | 8.1 |

From: www.concentric-medical.com

**Table 3.2** (ICD)-9-CM procedure code for i.v. lysis

| ICD-9 CM procedure codes | Additional notes |
|---|---|
| Patients with i.v. tPA injected at transfer hospital V 45.88 – status post administration of tPA (rtPA) in a different facility within the last 24 h prior to admission to current facility | First, code the primary diagnosis, the condition requiring tPA administration such as: acute cerebral infarction (433.0–433.9 with fifth digit 1, 434.0–434.9 with fifth digit 1) or acute myocardial infarction (410.00–410.92). The diagnosis code will indicate whether the lytic was administered for a stroke or an MI. |

From: www.concentric-medical.com

System. This code is specifically used for an endovascular approach. It includes the pre-cerebral vessels in the neck, such as the common carotid artery, and the cerebral (intracranial) vessels of the head, such as the middle cerebral artery. It applies to endovascular removal of obstruction from head and neck vessel(s), i.e.

• Endovascular embolectomy
• Endovascular thrombectomy of pre-cerebral and cerebral vessels
• Mechanical embolectomy or thrombectomy

Mechanical Thrombectomy/Embolectomy:

Medicare severity diagnosis related group (MS-DRG) assignment is based on a patient's principal diagnosis, primary procedure and secondary diagnoses. With acute ischemic stroke (occlusion with infarct) as the principal diagnosis and endovascular removal of an obstruction of head/neck vessels as the primary procedure, patients may be assigned to MS-DRG 23 or 24 (Table 3.1). Other MS-DRG assignments are possible if a different condition is designated as the principal diagnosis" (Table 3.2).

Similar updates and coding examples were provided by EV3-Covidien for Germany: "(Neuroradiologische) Gefäßinterventionen Beispiele aus der Praxis zur Kodierung im G-DRG System 2010" EV3.

## 3.3     Useful Links

### 3.3.1    Australia and New Zealand

- Government Health Department
- www.health.gov.au
- www.moh.govt.nz/moh.nsf
- Foundation of Research
- researchaustralia.org
- www.frst.govt.nz
- Science and Technology
- australia.gov.au/topics/science-and-technology
- www.morst.govt.nz
- www.sciencenewzealand.org
- Health Research Council
- www.nhmrc.gov.au
- www.hrc.govt.nz
- The National Stroke Foundation
- www.strokefoundation.com.au

### 3.3.2    United Kingdom

- Medical Research Council
- www.mrc.ac.uk/index.htm
- British Heart Foundation
- www.bhf.org.uk
- Department of Health, Stroke Network
- www.dh.gov.uk/en/index.htm
- www.uksrn.ac.uk
- CRUK
- www.cancerresearchuk.org
- Charitable organizations
- www.charity-commission.gov.uk
- www.charitychoice.co.uk/categorysearch.htm
- The stroke association
- www.stroke.org.uk
- Chest heart stroke Scotland
- www.chest.org.uk
- Different strokes (especially for younger stroke survivors)
- www.differentstrokes.co.uk
- Afasic
- www.afasic.org.uk

### 3.3.3   United States

• American Heart Association (AHA)
• www.americanheart.org

### 3.3.4   Others

• World Health Organization www.whosis/mort/profiles/en/index.html
• NICE www.nice.org.uk

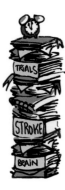

## Further Reading

http://www.improvement.nhs.uk/stroke/Unbundlingthestroketariff/tabid/259/Default. aspx. Last accessed 3 July 2011
Hospital Inpatient 2011 Medicare payment and policy update. Concentric medical. http:// www.concentric-medical.com/resources. Last accessed 3 July 2011
www.concentric-medical.com. Last accessed 3 July 2011

# Basic Milestones in Stroke Treatment

**4**

Key to a potentially good outcome of a stroke patient is the continuity of the treatment chain, which starts from stroke identification to treatment and further clinical management. In the USA, this is often referred to as the five "A's" in acute stroke management (Table 4.1).

Acute stroke management should be complemented with early supporting treatment and care. This includes early decompressive surgery in case of significant brain swelling, looking for and treating underlying causes of stroke (e.g., carotid stenosis), and optimization of management of vascular risk factors as well as early rehabilitation. Typically, this involves multiple disciplines such as specialist physicians, physiotherapists, occupational, speech, and language therapists, nurses, psychologists, and social workers. Effective rehabilitation is a critical part of recovery for stroke survivors and may help to return to independent living. There is a strong consensus among rehabilitation experts that rehabilitative therapy should begin in the acute-care hospital, immediately after the person's overall condition has been stabilized, often within 24–48 h after the stroke. It is thus an integral part of any stroke pathway and should be planned ahead of time.

Every hospital will differ regarding staff, equipment, expertise, and budget restraints. By identifying six important steps (Fig. 4.1) in the management of stroke, you will be able to structure your individual

**Table 4.1** The five "A's" in Acute Stroke Management

| | |
|---|---|
| **A**rrival | Emergency Medical Service (EMS) – Emergency Department (ED) – dedicated stroke space |
| **A**ctivation | Stroke pager-coordinate, ED, stroke neurologist, interventional neuroradiologist, neuroradiologist, X- ray technologist, etc. |
| **A**ssessment | Stroke neurologist |
| **A**dvanced imaging | Neuroradiologist |
| **A**dvance to treatment | Neurologist, interventional neuroradiologist (INR) |

I.Q. Grunwald et al., *How to set up an Acute Stroke Service*,
DOI 10.1007/978-3-642-21405-9_4, © Springer-Verlag Berlin Heidelberg 2012

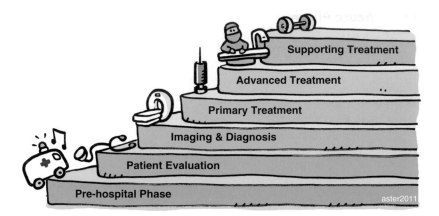

**Fig. 4.1** The six steps in stroke management

stroke pathway, tailored to your specific institutional possibilities and constraints. Once these steps have been identified, you can then address all the sub-aspects individually and identify the key people that need to be involved for each step.

Developing but also displaying such a work-breakdown structure will help you in dealing with the individual circumstances involved in each step.

So let us now look at the different steps that you will have to take when organizing an optimized stroke pathway through your clinical setting.

> **The major six steps in stroke management consist of:**
> 1. Pre-hospital phase with correct recognition of symptoms, timely, appropriate dispatch of the Emergency Medical Service (EMS) and patient as well as advance notification of the stroke team.
> 2. Patient evaluation and medical history.
> 3. Confirmation of the clinical suspicion "stroke" with modern imaging techniques leads to a diagnosis.
> 4. Primary treatment, e.g., lysis.
> 5. This can be complemented by advanced treatment, e.g., intervention, hypothermia, and supplemented by step six.
> 6. Supporting treatment such as early decompressive therapy and rehabilitation.

## 4.1     Acute Phase

### 4.1.1    Step 1 Pre-hospital Care: A Shortcut to Specialist Care

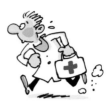

- Recognition of stroke symptoms
- Call of Emergency Medical Service
- Appropriate dispatch to stroke center
- Advance notification of the stroke team

Most time lost with stroke management is before the patient even gets to hospital. This underlines the importance of organizing pre-hospital care as well as public education to ensure adequate response and shortest transfer times. The aim here is to achieve timely, correct selection of patients with acute ischemic stroke and to appropriately initiate the rapid dispatch to a specialist center.

### 4.1.2    Step 2 Patient Evaluation

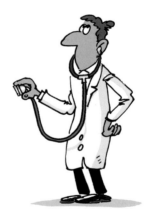

- Clinical examination
- Laboratory values
- Medical history

An essential step in ischemic stroke treatment consists of a clinical exami-nation, conventionally conducted by a neurologist or sometimes a stroke physician. It includes the taking of blood samples and the clinical history of the patient. Laboratory analyses and other tasks in this step can be greatly speeded up if assisted by a stroke nurse.

Clinical examination should determine severity of stroke and can already rule out possible differential diagnoses. Taking the patient's history should reveal possible risk factors or contraindications to further diagnosis or treat-ment. If, for example, the patient has a pacemaker, that would exclude him from

**4**

evaluation with magnetic resonance tomography (MRT). If there were a known severe allergy to iodinated contrast media, this would limit contrast enhanced imaging. Also, patients that have just recently undergone a major surgery or patients that are under warfarin have to be excluded from thrombolysis.

### 4.1.3   Step 3 Imaging and Diagnosis

- Imaging
- Patient triage

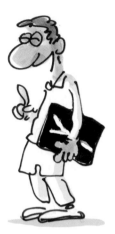

The third step, imaging, assists in the correct diagnosis of stroke and will greatly determine what, if any, further treatment options the patient might have. This will require an imaging technician as well as a neuro/radiologist who, ideally, will also be able to oversee suitability of the patient for any neuro-interventional stroke treatment. The combined expertise of the stroke physician, and the neuro/radiologist as well as the presence of the patient, will allow optimal patient selection regarding available resources and options.

### 4.1.4   Step 4 Primary Treatment

- i.v. lysis
- Nursing care

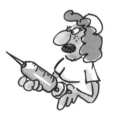

In most cases, the first treatment option will consist of intravenous thrombolysis, which will be administered, under ideal circumstances, while the patient is still in the scanner. The neurologist or stroke physician conventionally takes charge of this. In some centers, it will be the stroke nurse that administers lysis under supervision of the stroke physician.

In addition, the patient needs to be prepared and consented according to his/her further management. Ideally, for any further examinations and treatment, patients are undressed and have a urinary catheter placed.

While thrombolysis is running, especially in cases with major vessel occlusion, potential endovascular treatment can then be planned, and if necessary, the patient can be transferred to a specialist center.

### 4.1.5 Step 5 Advanced Treatment

- Endovascular treatment
- Neuroprotection

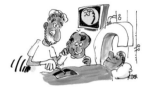

This stage will involve any interventional treatment of the patient either by intra-arterial thrombolysis or, more recently, by mechanical thrombectomy.

In many cases, endovascular treatment will primarily not be done under general anesthesia but done under sedation and local anesthesia. The main reasons for this are limited availability of anesthetic services and the resulting time delay for the patient. If, in your interventional stroke centers, ischemic stroke is already categorized as a "number one" emergency, equivalent to an emergency cesarean, initial intubation seems sensible. However, if this involves a significant delay in time, it might be more reasonable to begin with the angiographic procedure. Then, once the angiographic catheter is in place, with lytics being administered intra-arterially, intubation of the patient can take place – thus not causing additional time delay.

## 4.2 Post-acute Phase

### 4.2.1 Step 6 Post-acute Care: Placement

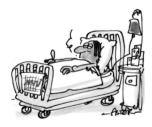

The next step, after the initial treatment of the patient, deals with correct placement of the patient. Obviously, if the patient was under general anesthesia, and especially in patients with basilar artery thrombosis, a ventilated bed should be available. In any case, acute stroke patients should be placed either on an intensive care unit or stroke unit.

## 4.2.2  Supporting Treatment and Aftercare

- Placement
- Timely clinical evaluation
- Decompressive therapy
- Underlying causes of stroke
- Management of vascular risk factors
- Organization of rehabilitation

During the first hours after the hyper-acute stage, monitoring and immaculate surveillance of the patient for possible complications is crucial. Patients can, for example, develop an intracranial bleed or, if they have suffered a significant stroke, will develop brain edema that can cause brain herniation and death.

These latter patients should be planned for timely clinical evaluation, before the expected rise in intracranial pressure. Younger patients that present with a significantly infarcted area in the middle cerebral artery or cerebellar territory in the morning have to be acutely considered for decompressive therapy in the evening. If they arrive in the evening, they can be planned for decompressive surgery the following morning.

Step 6 should also involve checking for the cause of the infarction, such as athero-embolic, cardio-embolic, lacunar stroke or stroke of another etiology. If an underlying cause is found, treatment should be initiated (stenting or carotid surgery, warfarin administration, or other conservative treatment such as anti-platelet aggregation drugs, statins, etc.). Finally, after optimization of management of vascular risk factors, transfer to a rehabilitation unit should follow. Here, patients and caregivers should be informed about possibilities and support available to manage life after stroke.

# Defining Your Priorities

# 5

This is a short exercise to reflect on the different areas of stroke service you can focus on. While ideally, each of the following aspects should be addressed, this might not be possible in your individual circumstances. Take a moment to write down which aspects of the stroke chain you can focus on and what you want to achieve. This will make it easier to "walk the six steps" that will define your own clinical pathway based on Chapter 4.

> Health care providers in all settings (hospital, private, nursing homes…) should be educated on the different treatments available for acute stroke as well as the critical time frames and should be able to identify patients at high risk for stroke.

Please define your goal:
e.g. *I will send out an information leaflet to local GPs explaining about our changes in stroke management and how they can be involved*

..............................................................................................

..............................................................................................

> Improvements in public education, pre-hospital care provider education, protocol development, triage and communication, and destination selection will make the difference between the implementation of advanced therapies and a lost opportunity.

Please define your goals regarding:
Public education, e.g. *write article for local newspaper*

..............................................................................................

..............................................................................................

I.Q. Grunwald et al., *How to set up an Acute Stroke Service*,
DOI 10.1007/978-3-642-21405-9_5, © Springer-Verlag Berlin Heidelberg 2012

**5**

Pre-hospital care provider education, e.g. *create information leaflet*

...............................................................................................................

...............................................................................................................

Stroke assessment protocol, co-operation with regional hospitals

...............................................................................................................

...............................................................................................................

Stroke pathway protocol

...............................................................................................................

...............................................................................................................

Patient triage – who and where?

...............................................................................................................

...............................................................................................................

Communication and contact person

...............................................................................................................

...............................................................................................................

Destination selection

...............................................................................................................

...............................................................................................................

Medical care for acute stroke starts within the pre-hospital setting. Already in 2008, the European Stroke Organization issued Guidelines for Management of Ischemic Stroke and Transient Ischemic Attack, which recommended, among others, the organization of pre-hospital and in-hospital pathways and systems for acute stroke patients.

Please define your goal:
e.g. *I will prepare pre-hospital and/or in-hospital pathways*

...............................................................................................................

...............................................................................................................

The first professional actor in this pathway is the Emergency Medical Services (EMS) provider, the link to the Hospital Emergency Department, who must be trained in the recognition of stroke and rapid transportation to the ED. EMS providers should know appropriate facilities for acute stroke patients and supply valuable information, such as stroke onset time and stroke symptoms.

Please define your goal:
e.g. *stroke evaluation form, in-hospital training, certification*

✎ .............................................................................................................

.............................................................................................................

The European Stroke Organization (ESO) further recommends that *"suspected stroke victims should be transported without delay to the nearest medical center with a stroke unit that can provide ultra-early treatment. In each community, a network of stroke units or, if stroke units are not yet available, a network of medical centers providing organized acute stroke care should be implemented and publicized to the general population, health professionals and the emergency transport systems."*

Each hospital should develop a treatment plan for patients with acute stroke that reflect its abilities and limitations. Hospitals without brain imaging facilities will not be able to treat patients with thrombolytic agents because "stroke mimics" such as intracranial hemorrhage cannot be excluded. Giving medication to dissolve the blood (lytics) to a patient with intracranial hemorrhage would most likely be fatal. Any other hospital with easy access to brain imaging facilities, radiologic expertise, and experienced stroke physicians should be able to treat and appropriately identify patients for intravenous therapy. In the absence of an active intensive care unit or neurosurgical expertise, it is then advised that patients treated with intravenous lytics should be transferred immediately after treatment has begun to a hospital with further facilities. It is likely that teleradiology will play an important role in rural hospitals.

Please define your goal:
e.g. *get/provide stroke expertise via telemedicine, set up co-operation with partner hospital for out-of-hour imaging*

✎ .............................................................................................................

.............................................................................................................

A stroke unit should be of sufficient size to provide specialist multidisciplinary care for the whole duration of hospital admission.

In areas where a stroke unit is not available or in remote rural areas, a stroke network with specialist support via telemedicine can be implemented.

Please define your goal:

*e.g. establish a dedicated stroke unit with x beds, engage intensive care unit (ICU)*

✎ ...........................................................................................................
...........................................................................................................

The ultimate goal is fast recognition and treatment of acute stroke. For this, it is essential to have a continuous chain of medical assistance from the pre-hospital setting to the patient's discharge from hospital. This should include the creation of stroke teams that are integrated in all the services involved in the care of acute stroke patients. You will be aware of the specialist services provided within your local and regional hospital setting. We would recommend you to now briefly outline a possible stroke chain so as to better oversee your goals:

Does your stroke service stop with initial stroke imaging and then involve transfer of the patient to a tertiary hospital? If it does, please underline those services *you* will actively be involved in.

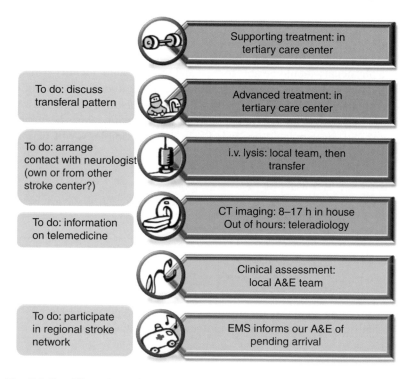

**Fig. 5.1** Possible pathway for a primary care hospital that wants to participate in an acute stroke service

Please follow the example below:

*Example*: *Primary Care Hospital with Limited Service*
   This is an example for a small, rural hospital without a dedicated Neurology Department. A CT scanner is available but there is no 24/7 support from Radiology or Neuroradiology. A technician conducts imaging out of hours.
   A possible pathway could look like the one on Fig. 5.1. The Emergency Medical Service (EMS) informs the Accident and Emergency Team of the pending arrival of a stroke patient. As no neurologist is available in the hospital clinical assessment is conducted by the Accident and Emergency Team. After 5pm images will be reported via teleradiology. A stroke neurologist (e.g. from a tertiary care center) can then initiate i.v. lysis and possible transfer of the patient to a center where interventional treatment and a stroke unit are available. Here supporting treatment like rehabilitation and work up of the patient history can start.

Here you can make notes for your own summary outline

✏ ...........................................................................................................................
............................................................................................................................
............................................................................................................................

# Walking the Steps and Defining Your Own Pathway and Goals on the Way

**6**

In order to define your specific goals, the necessary pathway from stroke diagnosis to treatment must be understood.

We will now guide you through the ultimate pathway a patient will undergo from first onset of symptoms to discharge from the stroke unit. Walking these steps with us will enable you to identify what is needed in the stroke set-up and what different options and alternatives you have. You can then tailor your stroke service according to your specific health care setting including the services you can offer and the specific requirements you want to fulfill.

Basically, the stroke pathway will again be divided into the six steps previously described:

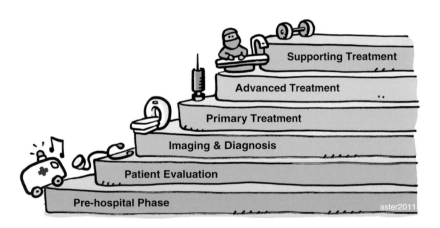

I.Q. Grunwald et al., *How to set up an Acute Stroke Service*,
DOI 10.1007/978-3-642-21405-9_6, © Springer-Verlag Berlin Heidelberg 2012

**6**

After each of the following sections, you are invited to take your own notes on:

> 1. Your specific goals per step
> 2. The team players you already have on this step
> 3. The team players you need to involve

## 6.1    Step 1: Pre-hospital Care

### 6.1.1   Notification of Pre-hospital Care Providers

Although a majority of people may recognize the symptoms of a heart attack, there is still a lack of understanding the signs and symptoms of stroke by a great number of patients, especially among the elderly, who are most at risk for stroke. Missing awareness of the signs and symptoms attributable to stroke may cause delayed medical attention and lead to irreversible damage to the brain. *Patient education* is therefore of utmost importance, whether it is delivered through the media or by primary health care providers. Using the Cincinnati Pre-hospital Stroke Scale or the Face Arm Speech Test (FAST) allows rapid identification and assessment of stroke. They are reliable and reproducible with a high inter-rater agreement among paramedics, the emergency department, and neurologists (see Appendix A.4 and A.5).

> Public and pre-hospital care provider education, development of protocols and pathways as well as patient triage, and destination selection will make the difference between the implementation of advanced therapies and a lost opportunity.

How can you improve public education?

✎ ......................................................................................................................
......................................................................................................................

The team players you have

✎ ......................................................................................................................
......................................................................................................................

The team players you want to involve

✎ ......................................................................................................................
......................................................................................................................

### 6.1.2   Notification of Pending Arrival of the Stroke Patient at the Hospital

As the possibility to treat stroke exists only for a limited amount of time, proper initial diagnosis of the patient is necessary. Even a short delay in the patients' arrival and delivery of care will significantly affect any potential for good outcome.

Considering the fact that a stroke patient will lose about two million brain cells per minute of delayed treatment, every measure that leads to early planning and activation of the acute stroke chain will ultimately translate into improved outcomes. For this, it is vital that the emergency stroke service system is integrated within the stroke chain.

In acute stroke, the ambulance team and pre-hospital care providers can significantly shorten the time between symptom onsets and definite therapy by *advanced notification of the stroke team.*

> Pre-hospital care providers are critical in the stroke pathway. Here, stroke should first be identified and the proper cascade initiated.
>
> In ideal circumstances, the ambulance team and pre-hospital care providers will be the first to set into motion the stroke team via pre-arranged, advance notification.
>
> This can dramatically diminish the time from hospital arrival to definite stroke intervention.

Special training and education for providers to recognize stroke might be necessary, but if the pre-hospital care providers are supplied with screening tools, they can accurately make a presumptive diagnosis of acute stroke. The *National Institute of Health Stroke Scale* (NIHSS), for example, is a standardized scale with little inter-rater variability that can assess the clinical severity of stroke (Appendix A.3).

In any case, pre-hospital care providers should be able to inform the stroke team already during transportation of the pending arrival of a patient potentially suffering from an acute stroke. The stroke team can then efficiently receive the patient and plan treatment.

How can you improve your pre-hospital emergency stroke service?
- *e.g. Provide training to ambulance staff*
- *e.g. Provide screening protocols and tools*
- *e.g. Establish contact person*

✎ ............................................................................................................

............................................................................................................

The team players you currently have

✎ ............................................................................................................

............................................................................................................

The team players you want to involve

✎ ............................................................................................................

............................................................................................................

**6**

## 6.2    Step 2: Patient Evaluation

After stroke onset, time is the most important factor, especially the first minutes and hours. As in any acute scenario, a patient with acute stroke must first be stabilized, which involves assessment of airway, breathing, and circulation (ABC). However, only a few stroke patients will present with an immediate life-threatening condition, but many will have severe impairments.

After the emergency assessment, a neurologist should perform a targeted neurological examination. This should be supplemented, if possible, by medical history, with particular focus on onset of the disease and on possible contraindications for thrombolysis. Imaging is essential to rule out stroke mimics such as hemorrhage or tumor, and a skilled interpretation of the results of CT and/or MRI scanning is essential for the best choice of treatment. This is the reason why some stroke teams will now arrange to meet with the patient in the imaging department (Walter et al. 2011).

> It has proven time effective for the stroke team to meet the patient at the point of imaging, e.g., CT as after stabilization and evaluation of the patient, imaging data will direct the pathways for further treatment.

Where will the patient arrive? *e.g Neuroradiology, Radiology, A&E?*

........................................................................................................

........................................................................................................

The team players you have

........................................................................................................

........................................................................................................

The team players you want to involve

........................................................................................................

........................................................................................................

Within the appropriate time window, i.v. lysis is the most common option for stroke treatment. Until a patient is clearly excluded from any thrombolytic or endovascular intervention, the emergency cascade should be kept in motion. Standardized neurological evaluation with the NIHSS stroke scale (Appendix A.3) can confirm and quantify the extent of stroke and monitor outcome. It also allows for accurate reassessment.

In your service, who will evaluate the patient?
Who will conduct a neurological examination?
Who will get the patient's history?

What standardized documentation is used?

✎ .......................................................................................................

.......................................................................................................

The team players you have?

✎ .......................................................................................................

.......................................................................................................

The team players you want to involve

✎ .......................................................................................................

.......................................................................................................

Rapid clinical evaluation and image interpretation will make the difference between potential eligibility for acute therapy and automatic exclusion based on time. This will only function if clear stroke care pathways have been defined. The consequence is that in the initial management steps, the coordination of patient care must focus on speedy evaluation and diagnostic testing.

## 6.2.1    Patients with Transient Ischemic Attack (TIA)

"TIAs" represent a brief episode of neurologic dysfunction caused by focal brain ischemia. The symptoms typically last less than 1 hour and usually present a significant warning of imminent ischemic stroke. The role of the stroke team here is:

1. To identify the possibility of a TIA
2. To exclude underlying causes such as carotid stenosis

The aim is to reduce future risk of stroke and to prevent ischemic stroke, e.g., via the administration of antiplatelet or antithrombotic agents, treatment of intra- and extracranial stenosis. A first step here is the placement of the patient in an appropriate unit to facilitate monitoring and to complete the evaluation.

It is important to perceive that a TIA is also a stroke and a neurological emergency. The placement of the patient with a TIA should be no different from that of a patient with more critical status. It can be compared to the patient with unstable angina. Current data clearly suggest that these patients need emergency evaluation to prevent recurrent stroke.

TIAs represent a significant warning of potentially impending stroke.

The main reason that patients do not receive the aggressive evaluation necessary is the fact that symptoms will often have resolved by the time the patient arrives. Given the known morbidity of TIAs, few, if any, patients with TIA should be discharged from the emergency department before evaluation of the cause of transient cerebral ischemia and the initiation of a subsequent treatment. Emergency physicians would not hesitate to admit a patient with unstable angina, even if the next day follow-up and testing as an outpatient could be obtained. Yet, this is exactly what is done for stroke patients with a similar disease but in a different organ. Thus, ideally, the emergency stroke team will initiate the evaluation of those patients with TIA beyond a baseline CT and start further treatment.

Based on the known data, it is not acceptable to wait for rapid outpatient evaluation and diagnosis of a patient's carotid stenosis. In an advanced stroke service, these patients should be observed in a unit with clinical protocols for diagnostic testing, carotid duplex, and echocardiography.

Who will evaluate the TIA patient?

..................................................................................................

..................................................................................................

Where will a TIA patient be placed?

..................................................................................................

..................................................................................................

The team players you have

..................................................................................................

..................................................................................................

The team players you want to involve

..................................................................................................

..................................................................................................

## 6.3    Step 3: Imaging and Diagnosis

### 6.3.1    How to Diagnose Stroke

The first question to be answered is whether the patient's symptoms are related to an ischemic stroke.

As seizures, intracranial hemorrhage, hypoglycemia, migraine and tumors can mimic stroke symptoms, the diagnosis of stroke is made by taking a careful history, performing a neurological examination, and confirming the clinical diagnosis with an appropriate imaging study. The techniques available include computer tomography (CT) and magnetic resonance imaging (MRI).

Choosing between one and the other will involve considerations on availability, speed, and sensitivity to detect stroke.

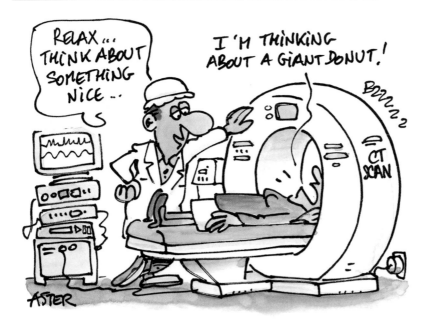

What imaging modality do I have?

✐ ....................................................................................................
....................................................................................................

What protocol will be used?

✐ ....................................................................................................
....................................................................................................

The team players and scanners you have

✐ ....................................................................................................
....................................................................................................

The team players you want to involve

✐ ....................................................................................................
....................................................................................................

## 6.3.2 Understanding Advantages and Limitations of Imaging Modalities

### 6.3.2.1 Computer Tomography (CT)

While non-enhanced head computed tomography (CT) is an excellent means to exclude blood and is important in the follow-up of the evolution of stroke, it also has certain limitations. Mainly, that it takes considerable time before the infarcted tissue becomes visible on the image and can be identified as a "darker," hypodense stroke area. In fact, in most cases, during the first

1–4 hours of stroke onset, the CT scan is normal, and even the few characteristic "early signs" that, in general, require the trained eye of a stroke experienced neuroradiologist, are absent. These early signs include the hyperdense middle cerebral artery sign, loss of the insular ribbon, as well as effacement of the sulci. Another limitation is that computer tomography is insensitive to small areas of infarction, especially in the posterior fossa.

However, due to its easy availability and rapid use, and as it already provides the key information necessary for hyperacute thrombolysis, namely – presence or absence of hemorrhage – CT is a frequently used and valuable diagnostic tool.

*Example 1: Non-contrast Enhanced CT* (Fig. 6.1).

Non-enhanced cerebral CT can detect blood and infarcted tissue. In this case CT could exclude blood but showed a hypodense (dark), infarcted area in the left frontal middle cerebral artery (MCA) territory.

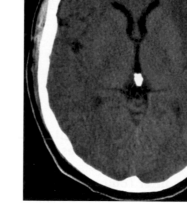

**Fig. 6.1** Non-contrast enhanced CT image of a left hemispheric stroke in the territory of the left frontal middle cerebral artery (*MCA*) branch. The darker, hypodense area represents a demarcated ischemic area that is presumed "dead"

**Fig. 6.2** In this case, the patient has a short but high grade stenosis of the right internal carotid artery just after the carotid bifurcation

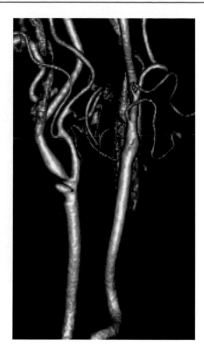

*Example 2*: *CT-Angiography*

CT-angiography is used to delineate the vessel anatomy. It can show an occlusion or even high-grade stenosis of intra- and extracranial vessels. CT-angiography requires the injection of contrast agent. It is very useful in the acute phase of stroke, not only to demonstrate the anatomy but also collateral flow (Fig. 6.2).

*Example 3*: *CT-Perfusion*

CT-perfusion studies can delineate the region of decreased cerebral blood flow. This is important to determine the penumbra, the amount of tissue that is likely going to die if the vessel is not rapidly reopened. If the area of decreased cerebral blood flow is the same area that has decreased cerebral blood volume, this is the area that will typically infarct and that cannot be saved anymore. If, however, the area of decreased cerebral blood volume is small compared to the area of brain that has decreased cerebral blood flow, successful reperfusion treatment here can then prevent further infarction (Fig. 6.3).

**Fig. 6.3** CT-perfusion: CT-perfusion scan showing a left-sided underperfused area (*black and dark blue*) involving the internal capsule and thalamus

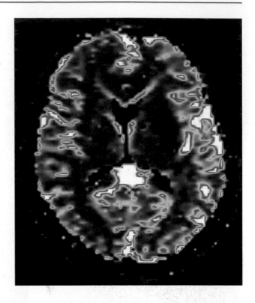

### 6.3.2.2  Magnetic Resonance Imaging (MRI)

Magnetic resonance imaging has contributed greatly to the diagnosis and management of acute stroke. Although not as readily available, many leading stroke centers are using MR imaging as the imaging method of choice, especially if interventional treatment options are considered. Main advantages are that the diffusion-weighted image sequence is sensitive to ischemia within minutes of the onset of symptoms (compared to plain CT, which will only show imaging signs of stroke after several hours) (Fig. 6.4).

MR is superior when the diagnosis is questionable and has been shown excellent for identifying small strokes. With the help of perfusion-weighted

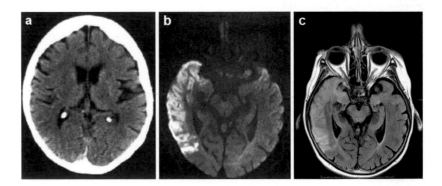

**Fig. 6.4** Patient with 4-h history of left-sided hemiparesis. While the CT image (**a**) only shows subtle changes, DWI (**b**) can demonstrate the fresh ischemic lesions within minutes. A FLAIR sequence (**c**) also reveals the right-sided infarct. This is also the sequence used to exclude any fresh hemorrhage on magnetic resonance imaging

MRI (PWI) it is possible to detect areas of the brain that are underperfused, i.e., do not get sufficient supply, but are still salvageable.

This penumbra is the area of brain where, without any further treatment, cell death will occur. The PWI/DWI mismatch region, defined as the difference in volume of tissue between the smaller diffusion lesion and the larger perfusion deficit, approximately corresponds to the ischemic penumbra and is the area that can profit most from early recanalization (Figs. 6.5 and 6.6).

If no mismatch is present, we presume that there is no relevant tissue at risk (penumbra). This means that a patient is unlikely to profit from interventional treatment.

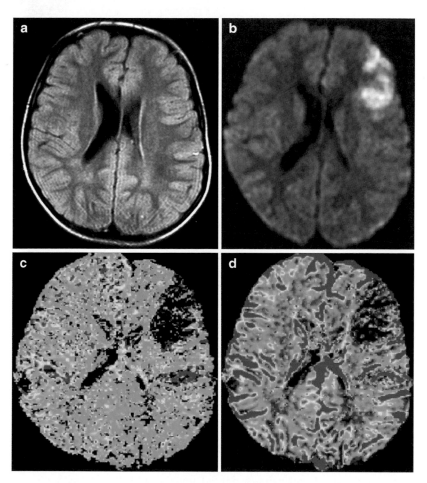

**Fig. 6.5** FLAIR imaging is normal, (**a**) the stroke sensitive DWI sequence (**b**) reveals a fresh ischemic lesion in the left frontal middle cerebral artery territory. Perfusion images (PWI) (**c**, mMTT; **d**, rCBV) show that there is no "mismatch" between the presumed irreversibly damaged brain area (as seen on DWI) and the underperfused PWI area

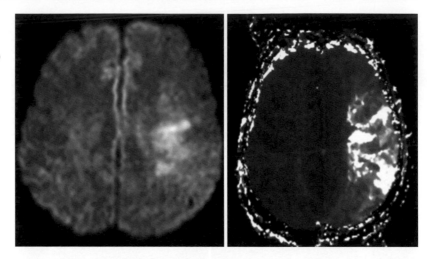

**Fig. 6.6** Mismatch. While the ischemic core on diffusion-weighted imaging (*DWI*) is only small, perfusion-weighted imaging (*PWI*) demonstrates a complete middle cerebral artery (*MCA*) territory involvement

*Example for "no mismatch"*

Figure 6.5 gives an example of a young patient who developed right-sided symptoms of stroke. While FLAIR imaging is normal, (**a**) the stroke sensitive DWI sequence (**b**) reveals a fresh ischemic lesion in the left frontal middle cerebral artery territory. Perfusion images (PWI) (**c**, mMTT; **d**, rCBV) show that there is no "mismatch" between the presumed irreversibly damaged brain area (as seen on DWI) and the underperfused PWI area. As no significant amount of salvageable tissue remained, no lysis was started.

In cases where a significant mismatch (discrepancy between infarcted tissue and underperfused area) is present, the patient is likely to profit from further therapy.

*Example for mismatch*

In Fig. 6.6 the patient arrived at the hospital 1 hour after stroke onset. While the ischemic core on diffusion-weighted imaging (*DWI*) was only small, perfusion-weighted imaging (*PWI*) demonstrated a complete middle cerebral artery (*MCA*) territory involvement. This patient improved significantly after thrombolysis.

This Mismatch method is now seen as the best way to predict which patients will most likely benefit from treatment and also which patients will tolerate a longer time window for any reperfusion therapy.

More information about "mismatch" can be found in Chap. 1.

Magnetic resonance angiography can also show a patient's extracranial and intracranial large vessels.

Depending on technique, this examination can be done with or without contrast agent (Fig. 6.7).

### 6.3.2.3  Digital Subtraction Angiography (DSA)

For specific questions, e.g., when obstruction or dissection of a large vessel is suspected, digital subtraction angiography (DSA) may become relevant, especially where intra-arterial treatment options are available. Digital subtraction angiography is still considered as the gold standard for visualization of extra- and intracranial vessels. This, however, requires specialized equipment and, for subsequent interventional procedures, interventional neuroradiologists. Due to the recent success of endovascular stroke devices, there has been a shift in stroke treatment with focus on endovascular, intra-arterial therapies that are now also often used as a first line treatment (Fig. 6.8).

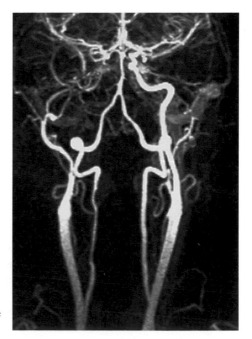

**Fig. 6.7** This contrast-enhanced MR angiography (*CE-MRA*) demonstrates a complete occlusion of the right carotid artery. The intracranial vessels on the right side are filled via the left carotid artery

**Fig. 6.8** DSA image: a contrast injection into the left common carotid artery reveals a high grade stenosis of the internal carotid artery

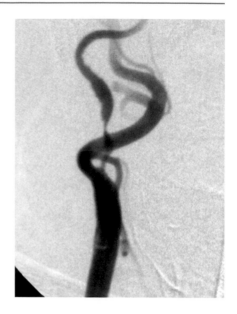

The increasing acceptance of endovascular neuro-procedures has recently led to the introduction of interventional angiography machines that can perform not only CT (Dyna-CT) but also CT-perfusion (Dyna-perfusion) scans, while the patient is on the angiography table. Until now these are, however, only available in a few acute stroke centers around the world, but the availability of flat detector (FD) Dyna-perfusion might represent the future in modern stroke imaging and treatment.

### 6.3.2.4 Multimodal Imaging
Multimodal neuro-imaging means that more than one imaging technique is used in order to gain different kinds of information about the brain parenchyma and vessels.

The evolution of multimodal neuro-imaging has revolutionized not only diagnoses but also management of stroke and should be the standard in any advanced stroke service.

**Why use multimodal imaging techniques?**

If the only question to be answered were:

"Is there a bleed in the brain?" then a non-contrast CT would clearly do the job.

In a modern stroke service, however, expectations toward imaging will be higher and should respond to the following questions:

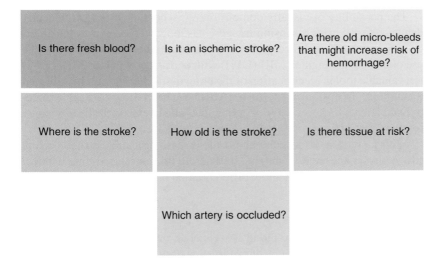

Nowadays, with modern imaging available, this information can be rapidly obtained within 5–20 min (Fig. 6.9).

Only multimodal imaging can answer all the above questions and thus enables patient selection based upon an individualized, physiologic tissue clock rather than a fixed chronologic clock (Molina 2005).

The multimodal techniques will be able to indicate the degree of collateral circulation, which is the critical variable in eventual infarct sites. Patients with a good collateral circulation can keep a large area of the normal tissue viable for an extended period of time. On the other hand, patients with poor collaterals are less likely to do well – even with early recanalization.

| | CT | MR |
|---|---|---|
| Is there fresh blood? Non contrast CT | CT<br>1 min | FLAIR<br>3 min |
| Is it an ischemic stroke? | Limited<br>sensitivity | DWI<br><1 min |
| Are there old micro-bleeds that could increase risk of hemorrhage? | – | T2*<br>< 2 min |
| Where is the stroke? | | DWI |
| How old is the stroke? | | ADC<br>< 2 min |
| Is there tissue at risk? | CTP<br>2 min | PWI<br>< 4 min |
| Which artery is occluded? | CTA<br>2 min | MRA<br>< 5 min |

**Fig. 6.9** This table lists how the different imaging modalities MRI and CT can be used in stroke diagnostic. (*CT* = computed tomography, *FLAIR* = fluid attenuated inversion recovery, *DWI* = diffusion weighted imaging, *T2\* MRI* = T2 star weighted imaging, *CTP* = perfusion-weighted imaging, *ADC* = apparent diffusion coefficient, *CTA* = CT angiography, *MRA* = MR angiography, *PWI* = perfusion-weighted imaging)

6

The possibility of visually demonstrating ischemic but not permanently damaged tissue using perfusion imaging has long been demonstrated and is gaining more and more acceptance. The recent studies have shown that the use of diffusion-weighted MRI (DWI) with perfusion-weighted MRI (PWI) is a valuable tool in identification of the brain tissue that can still be salvaged (penumbra). Diffusion and perfusion MRI have been shown to enable selection of patients for specific types of therapies and to extend the time window for treatment options.

With increasing knowledge about the disease "ischemic stroke," many stroke physicians are now moving away from the constricted time window for treatment that does not allow differentiation between patients with good and scarce collateral supply.

- Imaging of the brain blood vessels is an integral part of the standard risk stratification algorithm that every stroke patient must undergo. The information that can be gained has essential implications, both immediate and long term.
- Since the cerebral vasculature is implicated so often in the pathogenic process, imaging of both arteries and veins becomes a crucial part in stroke categorization.
- In addition to the diagnoses of stroke, knowledge of the vessel anatomy, site of occlusion, collateral flow, and flow dynamics within the brain allows better planning of endovascular therapy.

### 6.3.3   Laboratory

The American Heart Association recommends complete blood count, including platelet count and measurements of partial thromboplastin time, prothrombin time, serum electrolytes as well as serum glucose level.

Other laboratory tests, such as cardiac enzymes, can later become necessary but are not essential for the acute treatment of ischemic stroke. Usually, these examinations are performed in the centralized hospital laboratory. With the aim to reduce time loss associated with sending samples to such centralized laboratory, small point-of-care laboratory systems have been investigated for possible reduction of analysis times.

With the latter, platelet count, leukocyte count, erythrocyte count, hemoglobin and hematocrit (e.g., PocH 100i, Sysmex, Hamburg, Germany), international normalized ratio and activated partial thromboplastin time (Hemochron Jr., ITC, Edison, NY, USA) and γ-glutamyltransferase, p-amylase, and glucose (Reflotron plus, Roche Diagnostics Mannheim, Germany) can be quantified as requested by current stroke management guideline (Adams et al. 2007; European Stroke Organization 2008; Boehringer 2009) (Fig. 6.10).

**Fig. 6.10** Small point-of-care laboratory systems are now available and greatly facilitate evaluation of patients in the acute setting, even at the emergency site

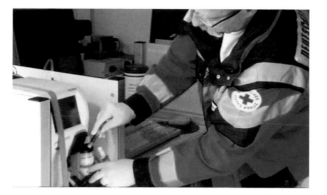

## 6.4    Step 4: Primary Stroke Treatment

Basically, the hyper-acute treatment within the first moments of arrival consists of supportive therapy, the administration of medication that can dissolve blood clots (lysis), and/or the direct recanalization of the vessel by endovascular means. The current treatment options, their rationale, and the level of evidence are listed underneath in "understanding current treatment options."

What treatment options can your hospital offer?

✎ ......................................................................................................
......................................................................................................

The team players you have

✎ ......................................................................................................
......................................................................................................

The team players you want to involve

✎ ......................................................................................................
......................................................................................................

### 6.4.1    Understanding Current Treatment Options

The successes, advantages, and risks of the various acute stroke therapies can be graded by their ability to recanalize and the ultimate test as determined by the clinical outcome.

Common scores and scales to evaluate recanalization are the TIMI and TICI scores. Outcome is usually graded by the NIHSS, Barthel, or mRS scale. These are listed in the Appendix.

Thrombolytic agents like rtPA have the ability to dissolve clot, thus reopening vessels and rescuing regions of brain otherwise destined for infarction. They can either be given intravenously or directly into the thrombus. However, time is of the essence. The time elapsed from symptom onset to reopening of the vessel is the surrogate marker for the degree of ischemic brain injury.

*Intravenous* tPA has long been shown effective within the 3-hours time window (Marler et al. 2000). A pooled analysis of three major clinical trials suggested that this time window could be extended to 4.5 hours (Hacke et al. 2004).

This was subsequently supported by the European study group, which demonstrated that i.v. tPA is also efficacious within a 3–4.5-hours time window (Hacke et al. 2008). However, although shown to be clinically effective, the licence for intravenous tPA is, at the moment, only within the first 3 hours, according to the present instructions for use. Yet, many hospitals administer rtPA within the prolonged temporal window of 4.5 hours – as off-label use.

Catheter-delivered thrombolytic agents directly address the *intra-arterial* clot. Promising results of i.a. recanalization trials have demonstrated benefit up to and beyond 6 hours after stroke onset (Furlan et al. 1999).

In a trial looking at occlusions in the middle cerebral artery (MCA), intra-arterial lysis was shown to be more effective than intravenous lysis (Mattle 2007).

In addition to lytics, *endovascular devices* can be used to recanalize the vessels.

Unfortunately, special expertise and an angiography suite are necessary for intra-arterial recanalization, and this is rarely available in most community hospitals.

In these cases, starting intravenous lysis while transferring the patient to a specialized unit (*drip and ship technique*) to continue with intra-arterial recanalization (*bridging*) can prove effective (Fig. 6.11).

### 6.4.2   Intravenous Thrombolysis

In 1996, the United States Food and Drug Administration (FDA) approved intravenous recombinant tissue plasminogen activator (i.v. rtPA) for the

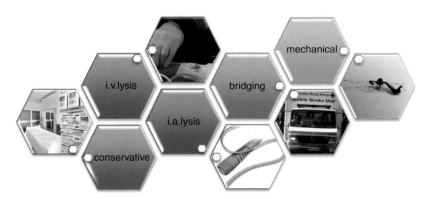

**Fig. 6.11** Current treatment options: next to a conservative treatment, current options include: intravenous lysis, intra-arterial lysis, bridging therapy, and mechanical recanalization

treatment of acute ischemic stroke based on two randomized trials comparing the effects of i.v. rtPA to placebo in patients treated within 3 hours of stroke symptom onset (NINDS rtPA Stroke Study Group 1995).

These trials showed that intravenous rtPA improved 3-month outcome if administered within the 3-hours *"critical window of opportunity"* from stroke symptom onset. The ECASS III (Hacke et al. 2008) study extended the time window from symptom onset to thrombolytic drug administration from 3 to 4.5 hours. Results were confirmed in a "real world" setting, reaching even better results than in the ECASS III study (Wahlgren et al. 2008). Approval, as mentioned above, is however still limited to the 3-hours time window.

Beyond rtPA, other thrombolytics have been studied to push the upper limits of treatment time window while simultaneously attempting to limit the risks of hemorrhagic transformation using multimodal scanning technology to determine the size of the ischemic penumbra. One such agent is desmoteplase, which is made from bat venom and is a longer acting thrombolytic with greater fibrin specificity than rtPA.

*NINDS Study*
The National Institute of Neurological Disorders and Stroke study demonstrated significant clinical benefit for the treated patients with an acceptable risk of ICH.

Six hundred and twenty-four patients with ischemic stroke were treated with placebo or rtPA (0.9 mg/kg i.v., maximum 90 mg) within 3 hours of symptom onset, with approximately one half treated within 90 minutes.

The study was conducted in two parts.

Part I: The primary endpoint was neurological improvement at 24 hours, as indicated by complete neurological recovery or an improvement of ≥4 points on the NIHSS.

Part II: The primary endpoint was a global odds ratio for a favorable outcome, defined as complete or nearly complete neurological recovery 3 months after stroke. Favorable outcomes were achieved in 31–50% of patients treated with rtPA, as compared with 20–38% of patients given placebo. The benefit was similar 1 year after stroke.

The major risk of treatment was symptomatic brain hemorrhage, which occurred in 6.4% of patients treated with rtPA and 0.6% of patients given placebo. However, the death rate in the two treatment groups was similar at 3 months (17% versus 20%) and 1 year (24% versus 28%).

Although the presence of edema or mass effect on baseline CT scan was associated with higher risk of symptomatic intracranial hemorrhage, a follow-up study demonstrated that the presence of early ischemic changes on CT scan was not associated with adverse outcome (NINDS rtPA Stroke Study Group 1995).

**6**

> *ECASS III*
> ECASS III showed that in 821 stroke patients, those allocated to i.v. rtPA administered up to 4.5 hours from symptom onset ($n=418$) were more likely to have a favorable outcome at 90 days as defined by a modified Rankin score of 0–1 (52.4% versus 45.2% for placebo; $p=0.04$). While mortality rates were not significantly different (7.7% versus 8.4%), intracranial hemorrhage was observed with a greater frequency in the treatment group (27.0% versus 17.6%; $p=0.001$) (Hacke et al. 2008).

### 6.4.2.1  Advantages and Disadvantages of Intravenous Lysis

rtPA has a narrow therapeutic time window and low efficacy in patients with large proximal artery occlusions or with severe deficits.

However, i.v. tPA is superior to conventional therapy (e.g., heparin or antiplatelet agents) and should be initiated immediately in eligible patients.

It can be given without much special expertise, is clearly beneficial in acute ischemic stroke, and requires minimal technology for patient selection (CT scan, laboratory).

Who will deliver i.v. thrombolysis?

........................................................................................................................

........................................................................................................................

Where will thrombolysis be given? *e.g. in scanner, in A&E?*

........................................................................................................................

........................................................................................................................

The team players you have

........................................................................................................................

........................................................................................................................

The team players you want to involve

........................................................................................................................

........................................................................................................................

## 6.5     Step 5: Advanced Stroke Treatment

### 6.5.1   Intra-arterial Thrombolysis

Large clot burden in vessels such as the internal carotid artery or basilar artery can often be resistant to thrombolytic therapy.

In an effort to increase recanalization rates and extend treatment availability to stroke patients and to reduce the potential for intracranial hemorrhage, intra-arterial (i.a.) lysis (delivering a lytic agent directly into the thrombus) was introduced.

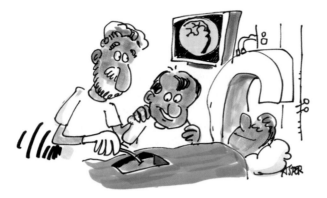

The PROACT II study (Furlan 1999) demonstrated a 15% absolute benefit in functional independence at 90 days using intra-arterial lysis 6 hours from symptom onset in patients with a middle cerebral artery occlusion. The study from Mattle et al. (Mattle et al. 2008) compared outcome after intra-arterial versus intravenous thrombolysis. Even though patients in the intra-arterial group were treated later, the outcome was still significantly better and mortality lower (4.7% versus 23%). It can thus be concluded that intra-arterial thrombolysis, at least in this specific group of patients, is superior to systemic intravenous lysis.

While few randomized trial data exists, intra-arterial lysis seems a viable option also for those who present in the 3–6-hours time window, independently of the degree of neurologic impairment. Most stroke centers agree that in basilar artery thrombosis, the high mortality of the untreated patients justifies intra-arterial thrombolysis, even at 12 hours or more after stroke onset. Successful outcomes with i.a. treatment have been demonstrated well beyond the traditional 3-hours time window.

*Advantages of Intra-arterial Thrombolysis Include*:
- Visualization of the actual vascular lesion is possible.
- Administration of smaller doses of thrombolytic medication reduces the risk of bleed.
- A lower dose of fibrinolytic agents can reach a higher concentration when injected directly into the thrombus as compared to a systemic infusion and is likely to produce a higher recanalization rate.
- The therapeutic window extends to 6 hours and probably longer (off-label use, please check instructions for use).
- Intra-arterial thrombolytics can be combined with mechanical clot disruption.
- Special expertise and an angiography suite are necessary.

**The Big Studies on Intra-arterial Lysis**
*PROACT II*
The Prolyse in Acute Cerebral Thromboembolism (PROACT) II study aimed to demonstrate that using intra-arterial lysis with prourokinase 6 hours from symptom onset in patients with a middle cerebral artery occlusion would be of benefit. One hundred and eighty patients with angiographically proven middle cerebral artery (MCA) occlusion were randomized in a 2:1 ratio to intra-arterial prourokinase or heparin control. The study showed a 15% absolute benefit in functional independence at 90 days (modified Rankin Scale 0–2) occurring to patients receiving treatment with prourokinase. Unfortunately, i.a. prourokinase did not receive FDA approval (Furlan 1999, Del Zoppo 1998).
*MELT*
The Japanese "middle cerebral artery embolism local fibrinolytic intervention trial" (MELT) aimed to determine the safety and clinical efficacy of intra-arterial infusion of urokinase in patients with stroke within 6 hours of onset. This randomized trial might have provided additional evidence for the efficacy of intra-arterial therapy but was stopped prematurely by the Independent Monitoring Committee after approval of i.v. rtPA on Japan. A total of 114 patients underwent randomization. Good clinical outcome (mRS 0–1) was more frequent in the urokinase group than in the randomized i.v. control group (42.1% versus 22.8%, $p = 0.045$). Although mRS 0–2 at 90 days was more frequent in the urokinase group (49.1% versus 38.6%), this did not reach a significant level ($p = 0.345$). However, there were significantly more patients with NIHSS 0 or 1 at 90 days in the UK group than the control group ($p = 0.017$). Randomized trial of intraarterial infusion of urokinase within 6 h of middle cerebral artery stroke: the middle cerebral artery embolism local fibrinolytic intervention trial (MELT) Japan (Ogawa et al. 2007).

Mattle et al. compared the outcome measures of intra-arterial versus intravenous thrombolysis for ischemic stroke in 112 patients. Two very similar groups of patients with middle cerebral artery (MCA) occlusion as detected by the hyperdense sign on computer tomography (CT) were assigned to intravenous plasminogen activator or intra-arterial urokinase within 3 (i.v.) or 6 hours (i.a.), respectively. Despite the fact that the mean time from symptom onset to treatment was longer (244 min) in the intra-arterial group than the intravenous group (156 min), patients in the intra-arterial group had a significantly better (mRS 0–2) outcome (53% versus 23%, $p < 0.001$). Furthermore, mortality in the intra-arterial group was lower ($n = 4$, 4.7%) compared to the intravenous group ($n = 13$, 23%; $p < 0.003$) (Mattle et al. 2008).

## 6.5.2  Intravenous Combined with Intra-arterial Thrombolysis

As special expertise and a catheter lab are necessary for intra-arterial recanalization, it is an option to start with intravenous lysis while transferring
the patient to a tertiary care center that can perform intra-arterial recanalization. Starting with i.v. lysis and continuing intra-arterially is called "bridging concept."

A trial of fundamental importance is the IMS II Trial (The IMS II Trial
Investigators 2007), which compared standard i.v. lysis versus combined
i.v./i.a. lysis (sometimes assisted with a micro-infusion catheter (EKOS)).
Outcomes were significantly better using the i.v./i.a. approach. IMS II also
confirmed again the correlation between successful recanalization and good
clinical outcome.

*IMS II Trial*
The IMS II Trial (Interventional Management of Stroke 2007) compared the combined i.v./i.a. lysis versus the standard i.v. lysis in
patients treated within the 3-hours time window after symptom onset
compared to a historical placebo control (NINDS) (NINDS rtPA
Stroke Study Group 1995). Two-thirds of the i.v. rtPA standard dose
were administered (0.6 mg/kg 15% of the dose as a bolus over 1 min
with the remainder administered over 30 min, up to 60 mg maximum). After angiography and in the presence of a persistent occlusion, an intervention was performed with intra-arterial therapy using
either the EKOS micro-infusion system (EKOS Corporation,
Bothell, WA, USA) or a standard microcatheter. Out of 3,602
screened patients, 81 patients were enrolled and treated (26 with
intravenous rtPA alone and 55 with i.v./i.a. intervention). Of the 55
patients, 19 were treated with a standard microcatheter, and in 36
cases, intra-arterial lysis was combined with EKOS micro-infusion
catheter. Up to 22 mg rtPA was administered intra-arterially over
2 hours or until thrombolysis was achieved. IMS II subjects had significantly better outcomes at 3 months than NINDS placebo treated
subjects for all endpoints (OR > or = 2.7) and better outcomes than
NINDS rtPA treated subjects as measured by the Barthel Index and
Global Test Statistic. IMS II also provided evidence that the EKOS
Primo sonography microcatheter exhibits a trend toward improved
recanalization of the occlusion as compared with a standard micro-
catheter and again confirmed the correlation between recanalization
and reperfusion with good clinical outcome and reduced mortality
(The IMS II Trial Investigators 2007).

**6**

*IMS III Trial*
The randomized IMS III Trial, which started enrolment in 2006, compares the combined i.v./i.a. approach to the standard i.v. rtPA alone, within 3 hours of acute ischemic stroke onset. A secondary objective is to determine the cost-effectiveness of the combined i.v./i.a. approach as compared with the standard i.v. rtPA. It includes not only the EKOS and standard microcatheters but also the Concentric Merci retriever and the Penumbra System device as a potential option for clot removal in the i.v./i.a. paradigm.

*Lysis Does Not Always Work*
Current data suggest that more than 50% of patients who receive rtPA do not demonstrate a favorable clinical response (Schellinger et al. 2001). In fact, when intravenous therapy is used beyond the 3-hours time window, there is an inherent risk of intracranial bleeding and cerebral edema from reperfusion injuries. Especially, large intracranial thrombi can be resistant to thrombolytic treatment, emphasizing the need for therapeutic alternatives.

*Intravascular Thrombolysis Combined with Mechanical Thrombectomy*
Endovascular stroke interventions can combine the use of intra-arterial thrombolytics, mechanical embolectomy devices, and angioplasty (balloon dilatation) with or without stenting. These procedures were originally implemented in patients who were either refractory to or ineligible for intravenous rtPA but are now more and more used as a frontline treatment.

The designs of the devices vary between their individual engineering concepts and their approaches to the clot, proximally, distally, or by squashing the clot to the vessel wall to create a patent lumen.

The initial concern about the risk of vessel perforation, as the devices are navigated to the clot, seems to have been unfounded as neuro-interventionalists continue to demonstrate. Although a randomized trial is still pending, multiple safety and performance trials have been performed with the current devices with encouraging results and recanalization rates of >80% (Bose et al. 2008; The Penumbra Pivotal Stroke Trial Investigators 2009).

The recently published results of the RECANALISE study (Mazighi et al. 2009) showed that a combined i.v.–endovascular approach was associated with higher recanalization rates than i.v. lysis alone. Again, better clinical outcome was associated with successful recanalization.

*RECANALISE Study*
The RECANALISE study (Mazighi et al. 2009) showed that a combined i.v.–endovascular approach was associated with higher recanalization rates than i.v. alteplase alone in patients with acute stroke and confirmed arterial occlusion. Fifty-three patients were treated with this dual approach, and recanalization was achieved in

87% versus 52% of 107 patients in the i.v. group (adjusted relative risk [RR] 1.49, 95%; CI 1.21–1.84; $p = 0.0002$). Neurological improvement at 24 hours (NIHSS score of 0 or 1 or an improvement of 4 points) occurred in 60% versus 39%. Mortality rate (17%) at 90 days did not differ in both groups, and symptomatic intracranial hemorrhage occurred in 9% in the i.v.–endovascular group and in 11% in the i.v. group. Better clinical outcome was associated with recanalization.

### 6.5.3 Mechanical Thrombectomy

The evolutionary journey of mechanical thrombectomy devices has graduated from adjunctive rescue treatment to frontline therapy. Mechanical devices seem to achieve faster recanalization with higher recanalization rates and may be more efficient at coping with material resistant to enzymatic degradation. Also, mechanical thrombectomy with little or no thrombolytic agent is a key option for patients with contraindication to thrombolytics (e.g., recent surgery) or advanced time window.

In essence, recanalization using mechanical means can extend the therapeutic window and potentially reduce the number of bleeds that are frequently associated with thrombolytic therapy. Limitations of mechanical devices have been reported and attributed to vessel tortuosity, arterial stenosis, and inaccessibility of the thrombus due to its location and consistency.

*Advantages and Disadvantages of Mechanical Stroke Devices Include*:
- Longer time window
- Can be used without lytics
- High recanalization rate
- Low availability
- High cost
- Risks during intervention
- Radiation

#### 6.5.3.1 The Merci Clot Retriever
One of the first successful devices for intracranial clot retrieval was the Merci Clot Retriever (Concentric Medical, Inc; Mountain View, CA, USA). It is an intra-arterially delivered corkscrew-shaped flexible nitinol (nickel titanium) wire that traverses and ensnares the thrombus, which is then removed by traction. The Merci Clot Retriever was evaluated in two international multicenter prospective single arm trials (MERCI 1 and Multi-MERCI )(Gobin et al. 2004; Smith et al. 2006; Smith et al. 2005; Smith et al. 2008) and showed recanalization rates of 43% with the device

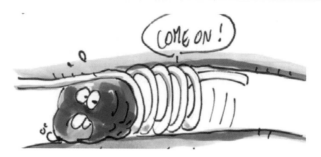

alone and a 64% recanalization rate with additional intra-arterial rtPA. The Multi-Merci study revealed a recanalization rate of 57.3% with the new generation retriever and 69.5% after adjunctive intra-arterial therapy.

### 6.5.3.2 The Phenox Clot Retriever

The Phenox Clot Retriever (Phenox GmbH; Essen, Germany) consists of three embodiments: pCR, CRC, and BONNET (Fig. 6.12). It consists of a self-expanding nitinol braiding with filaments passing through the interior to enlarge the surface area and enable better fixation of the thrombus mass.

While the BONNET resembles a stent, pCR and CRC basically resemble a pipe cleaner with perpendicularly oriented polyamide microfilaments.

In comparative in vitro studies, the Phenox Clot Retriever was able to filter micro- and macro-fragments that were formed during penetration and retrieval (Liebig et al. 2008).

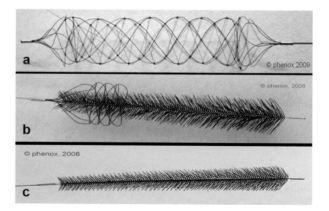

**Fig. 6.12** Showing the Phenox Clot Retriever. (**a**) The BONNET consists of a self-expanding nitinol braiding with polyamide filaments passing through the interior to enlarge the surface area and enable better fixation of the thrombus. The system can either be put distally to the thrombus or can be released into the thrombus. (**b**) The CRC is based on a fiber work of polyamide filaments whose lengths from the proximal to distal end increase. The CRC possesses an additional nitinol thread cage at the proximal end of its fiber brush. This nitinol cage gives it a higher radial range. (**c**) Phenox pCR is based on perpendicularly oriented polyamide microfilaments that create a dense palisade

### 6.5.3.3 The Penumbra System

The Penumbra System™ (Fig. 6.13) is a new generation of neuroembolectomy devices specifically designed to remove thrombi. The Penumbra System consists of reperfusion microcatheters that are connected to an aspiration pump (Fig. 6.14). A teardrop-shaped separator is advanced and retracted within the lumen of the reperfusion catheter to debulk the clot during aspiration.

**Fig. 6.13** The Penumbra System. A teardrop-shaped separator is advanced and retracted within the lumen of the reperfusion catheter to debulk the clot for ease of aspiration

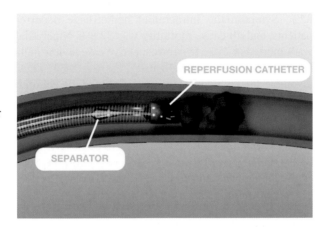

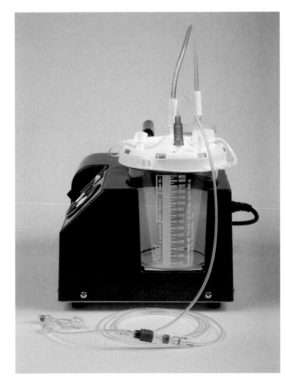

**Fig. 6.14** The Penumbra System aspiration pump. The Penumbra System is based on aspiration. A reperfusion microcatheter is connected to an aspiration pump through aspiration tubing generating a suction force of −700 mmHg

As a non-pharmacological tool, it has the potential of re-opening a vessel without the use of adjunctive thrombolytics, while offering dual options for recanalization via a single access platform. In addition, the system is designed to minimize the need to blindly penetrate into the occluded vascular segment since it operates from the proximal end of the clot.

The first feasibility Phase 1 Trial (Bose et al. 2008) showed a 100% revascularization rate (21 vessels). The Pivotal Phase 2 Trial (The Penumbra Pivotal Stroke Trial Investigators 2009) showed a recanalization rate of 82%. Symptomatic intracranial hemorrhage occurred in 11.2% of the patients, and all cause mortality was 32.8%. Ninety-day mRS score of 0–2 was reported in 25%. In a retrospective case review in patients treated by the Penumbra System, recanalization rate was 84%. Thus, it appears that the favorable safety and effectiveness profile of the Penumbra System observed in the pivotal trial can be extended to the "real world" setting.

*The Penumbra Pivotal Trial*

The Penumbra Pivotal Trial assessed the safety and effectiveness of the Penumbra System. It was a prospective, multicenter, single-arm study enrolling 125 patients with neurological deficits (NIHSS>8), within 8 hours of symptom onset, and an angiographically confirmed occlusion (TIMI grade 0 or 1) of a large intracranial vessel. Patients who presented within 3 hours from symptom onset had to be ineligible or refractory to rtPA therapy. The treated vessels of 81.6% were successfully revascularized to TIMI 2–3. There were 18 procedural events reported in 16 patients (12.8%), of which four events in three patients were considered serious (2.4%), but no events were adjudicated as related to the Penumbra Device. A total of 35 patients (28%) were found to have intracranial hemorrhage on 24-hours CT of which 14 (11.2%) were symptomatic. All cause mortality was 26.4% and 32.8%, respectively, at 30 and 90 days, and 25% of the patients had a 90-day mRS of <2. These results led to FDA approval.

*The Penumbra Post Trial*

In a retrospective case review study in 139 patients treated by the Penumbra System at seven centers in the USA and Europe, the device was found to successfully recanalize the target vessel in 84% of the cases with similar outcome and intracranial hemorrhage rates as the pivotal trial. In fact, 40% of the patients had achieved a mRS score of <2 at 90 days, which is a significantly higher rate than the rates reported earlier.

### 6.5.3.4 Intracranial Stenting in Acute Stroke

Recently, a self-expanding stent (Solitaire, Covidien, Mansfield, Massachusetts, USA) was used as a novel mechanical embolectomy device for

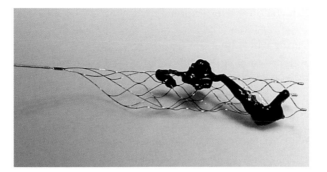

**Fig. 6.15**
Solitaire FR
revascularization
device. A
self-expanding
stent that can be
fully deployed and
then completely
retrieved. Not
approved for sale in
the USA

large artery occlusions (Fig. 6.15). The Solitaire offers the unique capability of being able to be fully deployed and then completely retrieved, if not detached. The stent is not yet approved for sale in USA but has received CE mark. A single-center, prospective, pilot study (Castaño et al. 2010) on 20 patients with an acute ischemic stroke attributable to a large artery occlusion of the anterior circulation, treated within the first 8 hours from symptoms onset showed successful revascularization (TICI 2b or 3) in 18 of 20 (90%) treated vessels. Forty-five percent of patients reached a modified Rankin Scale score of <2 at 3 months.

### 6.5.4  Future Studies

The ongoing registries of the Merci Clot Retriever and the Penumbra System as well as the Interventional Management of Stroke Trial III (IMS III) are currently collecting data on these emerging technologies.

Solitaire FR received a CE mark in July 2009, allowing for European sales. The Solitaire FR With the Intention For Thrombectomy study (SWIFT) began recruiting ischemic stroke patients in March 2010, intending to measure the safety and efficacy of the investigational device compared to results demonstrated in patients treated with a thrombectomy product already on the market and sold by Concentric Medical. Participants in the SWIFT study were to be measured at 30- and 90-day intervals after blocked arteries in the brain were recanalized and the clots removed.

Covidien is now hoping to gain regulatory approval in the USA for doctors to use the device to restore blood flow in patients during the first 8 hours after suffering a stroke. The company decided to stop enrolling new patients for the current study after conferring with members of a Data Safety Monitoring Board, a panel of independent experts that recommended that the company take the trial data to the FDA now, rather than wait for all 200 of the proposed participants in the study to be treated and tested. However, the company will continue follow-up care with patients already enrolled in the trial.

Can you offer interventional treatment?

✎ ...........................................................................................................

During which hours?

✎ ...........................................................................................................

Do you have an angiography suite?

✎ ...........................................................................................................

How are stroke devices paid for?

✎ ...........................................................................................................

Who sedates or anesthetizes the patient?

✎ ...........................................................................................................

Who organizes an interventional pathway including post-interventional
ICU bed?

✎ ...........................................................................................................

The team players you have

✎ ...........................................................................................................

The team players you want to involve *e.g. Neurology, Anesthesia,
Interventional Neuroradiology, Cathlab team, ICU team*

✎ ...........................................................................................................

## 6.6     Step 6: Post-acute Care/Supporting Treatment

### 6.6.1     Proper Placement of the Patient

Any patient with large ischemic stroke or after thrombolytic therapy should
be admitted to a dedicated stroke unit or an intensive care unit. Patients not
at a high risk of developing significant cerebral edema should ideally be
assigned to a monitored bed in a dedicated stroke unit (Fig. 6.16). If a stroke
unit does not exist, pre-destinated, monitored beds should be allocated to
where the acute stroke care pathway is well understood. If your hospital
does not meet these requirements, pre-arranged transfer agreements should
be in place to a facility that can accommodate the patient.

Who will organize a bed for the patient?

✎ ...........................................................................................................

How many ICU places can you provide?

✎ ...........................................................................................................

How big is the Stroke Unit?

✎ ...........................................................................................................

The team players you have

✎ ...........................................................................................................

The team players you want to involve

✎ ...........................................................................................................

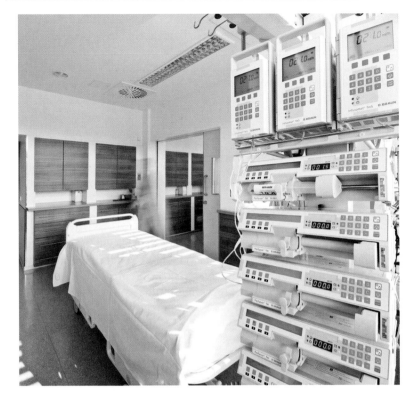

**Fig. 6.16**  Intensive care bed/stroke unit

## 6.6.2   Stroke Follow-up Imaging

Independent of the choice of treatment the patient received, the time span
that follows the initial evaluation and treatment will require further follow-
up of the stroke evolution. This is necessary to quickly adapt current treatment regimes. Especially in a scenario where clinical assessment may not
be easy or indeed impossible because of the need for deep sedation, imaging
becomes of paramount importance to plan any further therapy.

While MRI techniques have, over the last years, become very popular in
the emergency assessment of stroke (due to their versatility, accuracy,
thoroughness, and ability to provide significantly relevant additional information that has direct effect on the treatment), follow-up imaging for intracranial blood or hydrocephalus is still conventionally done with CT.

Currently, portable CT scanners that even allow CT-angiography and perfusion imaging are available and allow the study of critically ill patients on the ward,
without moving them from the intensive care unit. As infarcted tissue will develop
swelling, follow-up of the patient with malignant brain infarct is essential.

For further risk stratification, additional vascular imaging is necessary to
exclude underlying diseases, e.g., carotid stenosis.

Naturally, frequency and method of imaging will depend on the individual
case and must be guided by the specific needs of the clinical situation.

Who will initiate further vascular work up? Who will evaluate the patient on the ward for early changes caused by hemorrhage or brain swelling?

✐ ..............................................................................................................

..............................................................................................................

The team players you have

✐ ..............................................................................................................

..............................................................................................................

The team players you want to involve *e.g. ICU physician*

✐ ..............................................................................................................

..............................................................................................................

### 6.6.3   Decompressive Surgery

Brain edema can cause mass effect and compress adjacent brain structures. The rationale of decompressive surgery is to allow expansion of the edema, reduce intracranial pressure, and increase perfusion pressure. The aim is to preserve cerebral blood flow by preventing further compression of the collateral vessels.

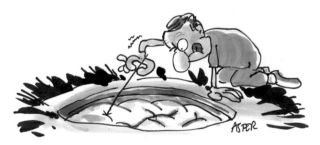

A malignant cerebral infarct is an infarct that involves the entire territory of the middle cerebral artery or internal carotid artery in one cerebral hemisphere. The mortality rate in these patients is, without surgery, very high. Patients that do survive will, in general, remain severely disabled and dependent. A widespread decompression with removal of part of the hemicranium as well as opening of the dura can be lifesaving, especially in the early course of the disease.

In space-occupying cerebellar infarction, decompressive surgery is considered the treatment of choice. Previous studies have shown that after this procedure, many patients, particularly the young ones, recover function more frequently than if they are not operated on (Mori et al. 2001; Schwab et al. 1998). Comatose patients with space-occupying cerebellar infarctions have a mortality rate of about 80% if treated conservatively.

Surgical, decompressive therapy in hemispheric space-occupying infarction was able to lower mortality from 80% to 30% without increasing the rate of severely disabled survivors. Early decompressive surgery within the first 24 hours after stroke onset could reduce mortality even more markedly (Smith et al. 2011).

There is now strong evidence from large meta-analyses of controlled trials to support the use of decompressive surgery for the treatment of cerebral edema in acute ischemic stroke. The HAMLET trial (The HAMLET trial 2009) started in September 2002 and assessed the effect of decompressive surgery *within 4 days* of the onset of symptoms on patients with space-occupying hemispheric infarction.

Sixty-four patients were randomized *within 4 days* of the onset of symptoms to surgical decompression followed by intensive care treatment ($n = 32$) or conservative treatment (consisting of either intensive care treatment or standard therapy on a stroke unit). The primary outcome measure was the modified Rankin Scale (mRS) score at 1 year. As could be expected, such late surgical decompression (*within 4 days* of the onset of symptoms) had no effect on the primary outcome measure.

However, in a meta-analysis of those patients in the DECIMAL (DEcompressive Craniectomy In MALignant middle cerebral artery infarction), DESTINY (DEcompressive Surgery for the Treatment of malignant INfarction of the middle cerebral arterY), and HAMLET trial, who were randomized within 48 hours of stroke onset, surgical decompression significantly reduced poor outcome.

So, it seems that surgical decompression can indeed reduce case fatality and poor outcome in patients with space-occupying infarctions who are treated within 48 hours of stroke onset. However, there is no evidence that this operation can still improve functional outcome when it is delayed as late as up to 96 hours after stroke onset. The decision to perform the operation should thus be timely and depend on the emphasis of patients and relatives attribute to survival and dependency. The operation should be performed before signs of herniation are present!

Can your hospital provide neurosurgical decompression within 48 hours or earlier?

✏️ ...........................................................................................................................

...........................................................................................................................

Where and how will patients be transferred?

✏️ ...........................................................................................................................

...........................................................................................................................

The team players you have

✏️ ...........................................................................................................................

...........................................................................................................................

The team players you want to involve

✏️ ...........................................................................................................................

...........................................................................................................................

Early surgical decompression of large infarctions can be a lifesaving measure.

**6**

**Abstract from the NICE Guidelines**
*Surgical Referral for Decompressive Hemicraniectomy*
People with middle cerebral artery infarction who meet all of the criteria below should be considered for decompressive hemicraniectomy. They should be referred within 24 hours of onset of symptoms and treated within a maximum of 48 hours.

- Aged 60 years or under.
- Clinical deficits suggestive of infarction in the territory of the middle cerebral artery, with a score on the National Institutes of Health Stroke Scale (NIHSS) of above 15.
- Decrease in the level of consciousness to give a score of 1 or more on item 1a of the NIHSS.
- Signs on CT of an infarct of at least 50% of the middle cerebral artery territory, with or without additional infarction in the territory of the anterior or posterior cerebral artery on the same side, or infarct volume greater than 145 cm³ as shown on diffusion-weighted MRI.
  - Appropriately trained professionals, skilled in neurological assessment, should monitor people who are referred for decompressive hemicraniectomy (NICE clinical guideline 2008).

**Stroke in Children**
Smith et al. present the history and outcome of ten children with malignant MCA infarction managed in pediatric neurology centers in North America and the UK. The authors concluded that decompressive hemicraniectomy can be lifesaving and that this procedure should be considered in children, as it is in adults (Smith 2011).

### 6.6.4   Rehabilitation

Most acute stroke patients will require rehabilitation services. The fastest recovery from a neurological deficit occurs during the first 3 months after the onset of stroke. It is thought though that active rehabilitation should continue as long as objective improvement in the neurological function is observed.

As already established in the Stroke Unit Trialists' Collaboration in 2002, rehabilitation services should consist of a multidisciplinary team including a physician, physiotherapist, speech therapist, occupational therapist, neuropsychologist, social worker, and nurse. Rehabilitation of a stroke victim should be started as soon as the patient is clinically stable. If the patient is unable to perform active training, passive methods can be used to prevent subsequent contractions.

Passive rehabilitation measures will also reduce the risk of bedsores and pneumonia, deep venous thrombosis, and pulmonary embolism.

Supporting a stroke victim in his/her social environment is important. Enabling the patient to keep up social contacts is perhaps the best opportunity to influence the patient's future quality of life.

In addition to national organizations involved in providing information to stroke survivors, the role of locally based self-help groups is important in supporting not only stroke victims, but also their carers.

Well-integrated social and medical care with case management programs may be one way to reduce admission to institutions and prevent functional decline.

Who will evaluate the patient?

✎ ...................................................................................................

Who will conduct rehabilitation?

✎ ...................................................................................................

Who will provide patients and carers with necessary information?

✎ ...................................................................................................

Where will this take place?

✎ ...................................................................................................

The team players you have

✎ ...................................................................................................

The team players you want to involve

✎ ...................................................................................................

Things you need to include in a complete stroke service:

A rehabilitation service that consists of a multidisciplinary team in a stroke unit (Level I evidence) that will:

- Provide evaluation of the patient for rehabilitation. If there is an indication for rehabilitation, this should be initiated as early as possible (Level I evidence).
- Provide stroke victims with a social network and guiding information. This includes intermittent follow-up by a family physician, outpatient rehabilitation services, and information on secondary stroke prevention and medication.

# References

Adams HP Jr, del Zoppo G, Alberts MJ et al (2007) Guidelines for the early management of adults with ischemic stroke: a guideline from the American Heart Association/ American Stroke Association Stroke Council, Clinical Cardiology Council, Cardiovascular Radiology and Intervention Council, and the Atherosclerotic Peripheral Vascular Disease and Quality of Care Outcomes in Research Interdisciplinary

Working Groups: The American Academy of Neurology affirms the value of this guideline as an educational tool for neurologists. Circulation 115:e478–e534

Boehringer (2009) Summary of product characteristics. Last updated on the eMC: 13/08/2009

Bose A, Henkes H, Alfke K et al (2008) The Penumbra System: a mechanical device for the treatment of acute stroke due to thromboembolism. AJNR Am J Neuroradiol 29:1409–1413

Castaño C, Dorado L, Guerrero C, Millán M, Gomis M, Perez de la Ossa N, Castellanos M, García MR, Domenech S, Dávalos A (2010) Mechanical thrombectomy with the Solitaire AB device in large artery occlusions of the anterior circulation: a pilot study. Stroke 41(8):1836–1840

Del Zoppo GJ, Higashida RT, Furlan AJ, Pessin MS, Rowley HA, Gent M (1998) PROACT investigators. PROACT: a phase II randomized trial of recombinant pro-urokinase by direct arterial delivery in acute middle cerebral artery stroke. Prolyse in Acute Cerebral Thromboembolism. Stroke 29:4–11

European Stroke Organization (ESO) Executive Committee: Collective Name: ESO Writing Committee (2008) Guidelines for management of ischaemic stroke and transient ischaemic attack 2008. Cerebrovasc Dis 25:457–507 and later revisions

Furlan A, Higashida R, Wechsler L et al (1999) Intra-arterial prourokinase for acute ischemic stroke. The PROACT II Study: a randomized controlled trial. JAMA 282:2003–2011

Gobin YP, Starkman S, Duckwiler GR, Grobelny T, Kidwell CS, Jahan R, Pile-Spellman J, Segal A, Vinuela F, Saer JL (2004) Merci 1: a phase 1 study of mechanical embolus removal in cerebral ischemia. Stroke 35:2848–2854

Hacke W, Donna G, Fieschi C et al (2004) Association of outcome with early stroke treatment: pooled analysis of ATLANTIS, ECASS, and NINDS rt-PA stroke trials. Lancet 363:768–774

Hacke W, Kaste M, Bluhmki E et al (2008) Thrombolysis with alteplase 3 to 4.5 hours after acute ischemic stroke. N Engl J Med 359:1317–1329

Hofmeijer J, Kappelle LJ, Algra A, Amelink GJ, van Gijn J, van der Worp HB; HAMLET investigators (2009) Surgical decompression for space-occupying cerebral infarction (the Hemicraniectomy After Middle Cerebral Artery infarction with Life-threatening Edema Trial [HAMLET]): a multicentre, open, randomised trial. Lancet Neurol 8(4):326–333. Epub 2009 Mar 5

Liebig T, Reinartz J, Hannes R, Miloslavski E, Henkes H (2008) Comparative in vitro study of five mechanical embolectomy systems: effectiveness of clot removal and risk of distal embolization. Neuroradiology 50:43–52

Marler JR, Tilley BC, Lu M et al (2000) Early stroke treatment associated with better outcome: the NINDS rt-PA Stroke Study. Neurology 55:1649–1655

Mattle H (2007) Intravenous or intra-arterial thrombolysis? It's time to find the right approach for the right patient. Stroke 38:2038–2040

Mattle HP, Arnold M, Georgiadis D, Baumann C, Nedeltchev K, Benninger D, Remonda L, von Budingen C, Diana A, Pangalu A, Schroth G, Baumgartner RW (2008) Comparison of intraarterial and intravenous thrombolysis for ischemic stroke with hyperdense middle cerebral artery sign. Stroke 39:379–383

Mazighi M, Serfaty JM, Labreuche J, Laissy JP, Meseguer E, Lavallee PC et al (2009) Comparison of intravenous alteplase with a combined intravenous-endovascular approach in patients with stroke and confirmed arterial occlusion (RECANALISE study): a prospective cohort study. Lancet Neurol 8:802–809

Molina C (2005) Extending reperfusion therapy for acute ischemic stroke: emerging pharmacological, mechanical, and imaging strategies. Stroke 36:2311–2320

Mori K, Aoki A, Yamamoto T, Horinaka N, Maeda M (2001) Aggressive decompressive surgery in patients with massive hemispheric embolic cerebral infarction associated with severe brain swelling. Acta Neurochir 143(5):483–491; discussion 491–492

NICE clinical guideline 68 (2008) Stroke. National Institute for Health and Clinical Excellence. http://www.nice.org.uk/nicemedia/live/12018/41331/41331.pdf. Last accessed 3.7.2011

NINDS rt-PA Stroke Study Group (1995) Tissue plasminogen activator for acute ischemic stroke. N Engl J Med 333:1581–1587

Ogawa A, Mori E, Minematsu K, Taki W, Takahashi A, Nemoto S, Miyamoto S, Sasaki M, Inoue T, MELT Japan Study Group (2007) Randomized trial of intraarterial infusion of urokinase within 6 hours of middle cerebral artery stroke: the middle cerebral artery embolism local fibrinolytic intervention trial (MELT) Japan. Stroke 38(10):2633–2639, Epub 2007 Aug 16

Schellinger PD, Fiebach JB, Jansen O et al (2001) Stroke magnetic resonance imaging within 6 hours after onset of hyperacute cerebral ischemia. Ann Neurol 49:460–469

Schwab S, Steiner T, Aschoff A, Schwarz S, Steiner HH, Jansen O, Hacke W (1998) Early hemicraniectomy in patients with complete middle cerebral artery infarction. Stroke 29(9):1888–1893

Smith WS, Sung G, Starkmann S, Saver JL, Kidwell CS, Gobin YP, Lutsep HL, Nesbit GM, Grobelny T, Rymer MM, Silverman IE, Higashida RT, Budzik RF, Marks MP (2005) Safety and efficacy of mechanical embolectomy in acute ischemic stroke: results of the MERCI trial. Stroke 36:1432–1438

Smith WS, Tsao JW, Billings ME, Johnston SC, Hemphill JC III, Bonovich DC, Dillon WP (2006) Prognostic significance of angiographically confirmed large vessel intracranial occlusion in patients presenting with acute brain ischemia. Neurocrit Care 4:14–17

Smith W, Sung G, Saver J, Budzik R, Duckwiler G, Liebeskind D, Lutsep H, Rymer M, Higashida R, Starkman S, Gobin P (2008) Mechanical thrombectomy for acute ischemic stroke. Final results of the multi Merci trial. Stroke 39:1205–1212

Smith SE, Kirkham FJ, deVeber G et al (2011) Outcome following decompressive craniectomy for malignant cerebral artery infarction in children. Dev Med Child Neurol 53:29–33. doi:10.1111/j.1469-8749.2010.03775.x

The IMS II Trial Investigators (2007) The interventional management of stroke (IMS) II study. Stroke 38:2127–2135

The Penumbra Pivotal Stroke Trial Investigators (2009) The Penumbra Pivotal Stroke Trial: safety and effectiveness of a new generation of mechanical devices for clot removal in intracranial large vessel occlusive disease. Stroke 40:2761–2768

Wahlgren N, Ahmed N, Davalos A, Hacke W, Millian M, Muir K, Roine RO, Toni D, Lees KR, SITS Investigators (2008) Thrombolysis with alteplase 3–4.5 h after acute ischaemic stroke (SITS-ISTR): an observational study. Lancet 372:1303–1309

Walter S, Kostopoulos P, Haass A, Lesmeister M, Grasu M, Grunwald I, Keller I, Helwig S, Becker C, Geisel J, Bertsch T, Kaffiné S, Leingärtner A, Papanagiotou P, Roth C, Liu Y, Reith W, Fassbender K (2011) Point-of-care laboratory halves door-to-therapy-decision time in acute stroke. Ann Neurol 69(3):581–586. doi:10.1002/ana.22355, Epub 2011 Mar 11

## Further Reading

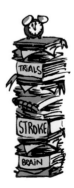

Jüttler E, Schwab S, Schmiedek P et al (2007) Decompressive surgery for the treatment of malignant infarction of the middle cerebral artery (DESTINY): a randomized, controlled trial. Stroke 38:2518–2525

SWIFT: http://www.clinicaltrials.gov/ct2/show/NCT01054560?term=Solitaire+FR+With+Intention+For+Thrombectomy&rank=1 last accessed 12.10.2011

Vahedi K (2009) Decompressive hemicraniectomy for malignant hemispheric infarction. Curr Treat Options Neurol 11(2):113–119

6

Vahedi K, Hofmeijer J, Juettler E et al (2007a) Early decompressive surgery in malignant infarction of the middle cerebral artery: a pooled analysis of three randomised controlled trials. Lancet Neurol 6:215–222

Vahedi K, Vicaut E, Mateo J et al (2007b) Sequential design, multicenter, randomized, controlled trial of early decompressive craniectomy in malignant middle cerebral artery infarction (DECIMAL trial). Stroke 38:2506–2517

Newswires: Covidien Product Showed Positive Results In Halted Study –CEO by Jon Kamp Published March 17, 2011 Dow Jones http://www.foxbusiness.com/industries/2011/03/17/covidien-product-showed-positive-results-halted-study-ceo/#ixzz1aamYG4Z2 last accessed 12.10.2011

# Bringing Your Goals into Shape 7

You have now covered the six crucial steps of the stroke pathway and have developed a vision of the service you could realistically provide. You will also have a broad overview of how the service could, in time, be expanded. Take a moment to review the notes you have taken previously in Chap. 5, as we will now ask you to draw a simple flow diagram (Fig. 7.2) of how you envision the treatment pathway of a patient with acute ischemic stroke that arrives at your hospital. Let us further assume that our patient is eligible for intravenous thrombolysis.

The flow diagram Fig. 7.1 should act as an example:

After initiation of the emergency chain, the ambulance team will inform a pre-assigned contact of the pending arrival of a potential stroke victim. In our case, the pre-arranged contact is the neurologist.

The neurologist will have gathered first vital information on the clinical situation and patient data and will thus be able to identify the best place to meet the patient (A&E, MRI, or CT scanner).

Informed by the neurologist or the stroke nurse, the team gathers at the point of imaging – in our case, the CT scanner.

A clinical evaluation can be conducted, and blood samples taken whilst the patient is awaiting the CT scan.

After contraindications for thrombolysis are excluded by the neurologist (clinical history and examination) and by the neuroradiologist (imaging), intravenous thrombolysis can be initiated at the site of imaging.

The patient is then transported to a dedicated stroke or ICU unit, depending on the clinical status. From here, further imaging will be initiated to monitor brain swelling and potential hemorrhage.

The neurosurgical contact can be consulted at this stage to pre-notify the team of a possible candidate for early decompressive therapy if a major stroke could not be prevented.

I.Q. Grunwald et al., *How to set up an Acute Stroke Service*,
DOI 10.1007/978-3-642-21405-9_7, © Springer-Verlag Berlin Heidelberg 2012

7

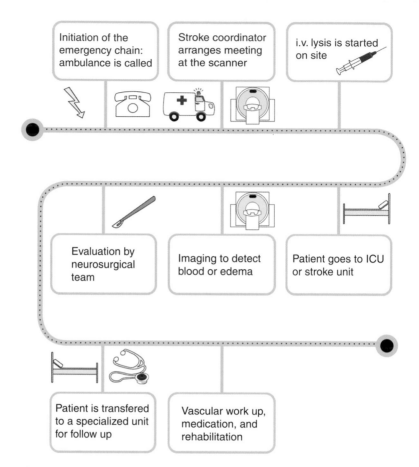

**Fig. 7.1** Flow diagram for an individual stroke pathway

Vascular workup to check for underlying risk factors and individual adjustment of medication will now follow.

Also, early rehabilitation can be planned in conjunction with physiotherapy.

Please draw your own diagram (Fig. 7.2) of how your patient will pass through your stroke pathway.

Consider who will be involved, how people are notified, where treatment is started, and where the patient will go after therapy.

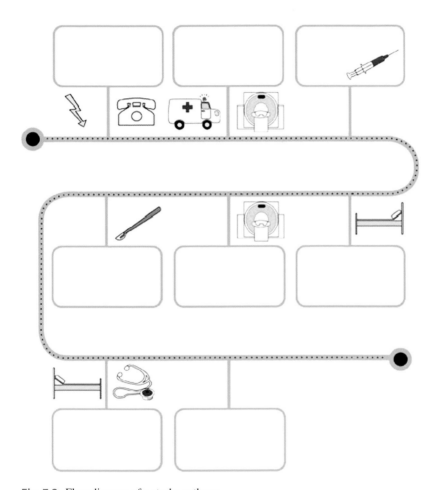

**Fig. 7.2** Flow diagram of a stroke pathway

# Examples of Treatment Pathways

# 8

## 8.1    Imaging Pathways

The key factors that will influence the outcome of a patient with acute ischemic stroke are the time it takes to reopen the vessel (from the stroke onset time), the patient's individual intracranial hemodynamics and inherent collateral flow, the viable tissue that is still left (penumbra), and the effectiveness of stoke treatment and intervention (Fig. 8.1). Imaging is useful in all these aspects.

Patients with strong collateral circulation, either directly via the circle of Willis or indirectly via collateral meningeal supply, can keep a larger area of tissue viable for an extended period of time than patients with limited collateral flow. Thus, a patient with poor collaterals is less likely to do well, even if early recanalization is achieved.

Nowadays, it is possible to examine the vascular anatomy by using CT-angiography (CTA) or MR-angiography (MRA). Also, it is possible to investigate the cerebral blood perfusion with both CT and MRI (CT-perfusion and MR-perfusion).

**Fig. 8.1** Factors that will influence outcome after ischemic stroke

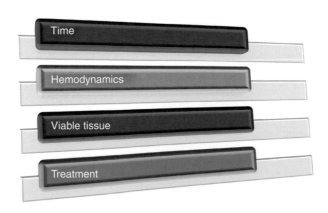

I.Q. Grunwald et al., *How to set up an Acute Stroke Service*,
DOI 10.1007/978-3-642-21405-9_8, © Springer-Verlag Berlin Heidelberg 2012

**8**

The imaging pathways supplied in this chapter all focus on patient selection based upon an individualized, physiological tissue clock rather than on a fixed time window. The concept is to assess the areas of the brain that are still viable, based on multimodal MRI and CT techniques.

This multimodal MRI and CT imaging, although only developed in the past decade, has by now secured its place in the diagnosis and treatment of acute stroke victims, as it helps to identify more accurately and rapidly those patients that are best suited for stroke treatment and intervention.

Modern clinical trials are now incorporating real time, multimodal imaging data into the patients' selection criteria and outcome analysis.

Both imaging modalities, MR and CT, are widely available and provide information on the state of the brain tissue, the vessels, and the perfusion of the brain tissue.

Some hospitals will have the ability to perform either or even both forms of imaging. To choose an appropriate pathway, many factors have to be taken into account. Your choice will depend on the clinical condition of the patient, the time since stroke onset, and, of course, the logistical constraint of your department. In addition, the decision will depend on the kind of stroke treatment the hospital is able to offer. For example, if the hospital can only provide a thrombolysis service and has no facility to perform further therapy such as intra-arterial lysis or thrombectomy, advanced imaging will often be useful but not essential.

Regardless of the stroke intervention you can offer, basic imaging is crucial in stroke management to differentiate the symptoms of acute ischemic stroke from those of acute hemorrhage.

For this, either MRI or CT can be used as alternate pathways.

### 8.1.1  Pathways Using Computer Tomography

Acute hemorrhage can quickly be excluded using computer tomography. It is however more difficult to detect the early signs of stroke using computer tomography. Early ischemic changes have been associated with a higher risk of intracranial hemorrhage when thrombolytic therapy is administered. This subsequently results in a poorer outcome after thrombolytic therapy for those patients where ischemic changes were already visible at the time of treatment.

Concerns have been raised about the ability of standard CT imaging to detect acute ischemic change.

The decision to begin thrombolytic therapy should therefore be made with the best information available. Using multimodal imaging (combining plain CT, angiography, and perfusion), CT-based imaging will also constitute a strong and valuable tool in both diagnosis and treatment of patients with cerebrovascular disease.

### 8.1.1.1  Plain Computer Tomography Only

When a patient presents with an acute neurological deficit, the differential diagnoses usually include ischemic stroke, hemorrhage, and transient ischemic attack (TIA). Other differentials are a mass lesion (either of traumatic, neoplastic, or infectious cause). As time is of the essence in ischemic stroke, CT should be used quickly to rule out some of the main contraindications for lytic therapy. An absolute contraindication for intravenous thrombolysis would be if the image showed any evidence of hemorrhage or a very large, well-established acute infarct.

If the patient has an acute ischemic stroke, a non-contrast enhanced CT scan (NE-CT) will, in the first hours:
- Either be normal (early stages of stroke)
- Show early signs of stroke or
- Show a different pathology (Fig. 8.2)

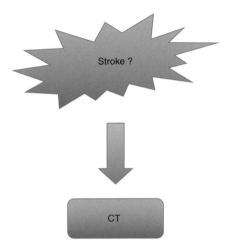

In the presence of blood, an alternate pathway will be initiated, which consists of vascular work up, neuro-intensive monitoring and care, and potentially neurosurgical intervention.

If the suspicion of an acute stroke is confirmed, the patient will then need to be assigned to one of three further management options. These are conventionally conservative management, intravenous lysis, or endovascular treatment (Fig. 8.3).

8

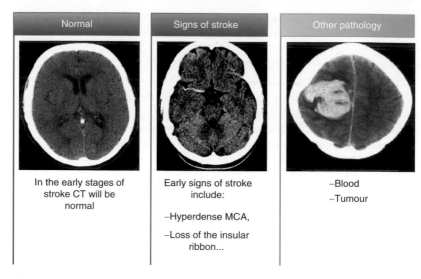

| Normal | Signs of stroke | Other pathology |
|---|---|---|
| In the early stages of stroke CT will be normal | Early signs of stroke include:<br><br>–Hyperdense MCA,<br><br>–Loss of the insular ribbon... | –Blood<br>–Tumour |

**Fig. 8.2** CT imaging in the early time window

**Fig. 8.3** The patient will be assigned to one of the three pathways: intravenous lysis, endovascular treatment, or conservative management

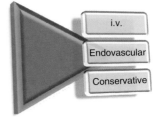

## 8.1.2   **Pathway Using Multimodal CT** (Fig. 8.4)

It is believed that a more sophisticated assessment of the hemodynamic issues in a patient, particularly the collateral flow, may influence stroke management and the choice of treatment for the individual patient. Utilizing multimodal CT provides more information and should not cause any significant delay for thrombolysis. It is also possible to start with intravenous therapy in eligible patients while the patient is still in the scanner, once hemorrhage or a mass lesion has been excluded.

The following pathways of stroke treatment, regardless of the modality used, will all include a multimodal approach as the standard imaging protocol in an acute stroke patient.

In the multimodal CT pathway a plain, non-contrast enhanced CT will be used to detect hemorrhage. If a bleed is found, the patient will then be assigned to further vascular work up (e.g., CT-angiography).

**CT-pathway**

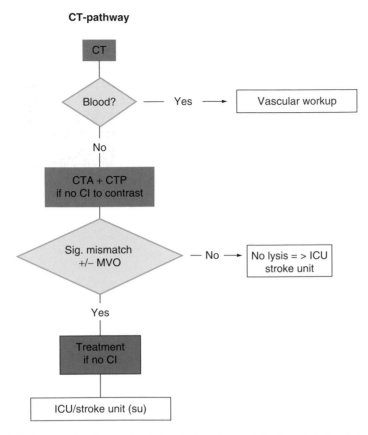

**Fig. 8.4** Suggested pathway using CT as the imaging modality in acute ischemic stroke: *SU* stroke unit, *ICU* intensive care unit, *MVO* major vessel occlusion, *CI* contraindication

If blood is excluded, CT-angiography (CTA) and CT-perfusion (CTP) will follow if the patient has no known contraindications (CI) to iodinated contrast media.

If a significant mismatch (tissue at risk) remains with or without evidence of a major vessel occlusion (MVO), this patient will be considered for further treatment, e.g., lysis or endovascular, once contraindications are excluded. Placement of the patient will then be on either a stroke unit (SU) or intensive care unit (ICU).

### 8.1.3   Combined CT and MRI Pathway (Fig. 8.5)

If you have MRI and CT in close proximity, the following pathway can prove beneficial. However, if your institution's CT and MRI scanners are in different locations, the optimal solution will obviously vary from hospital to hospital and from patient to patient. Any transfer can be time-consuming

8

and has to be weighed against the potential benefit to the patient. As scanning time on MRI scanners is usually not as freely available as on CT, some centers will already screen those patients that would potentially benefit most from MRI imaging (such as patients with posterior circulation stroke) and arrange with the ambulance service or emergency care provider that patients are brought to and met directly at the MR scanner.

The following imaging pathways aim to help develop the optimal solutions in order to maximize the number of good clinical outcomes in the acute stroke patient.

If you are in the fortunate position of having a CT and MRI system located in close proximity to each other, both imaging systems can be combined and used to complement each other (Fig. 8.5).

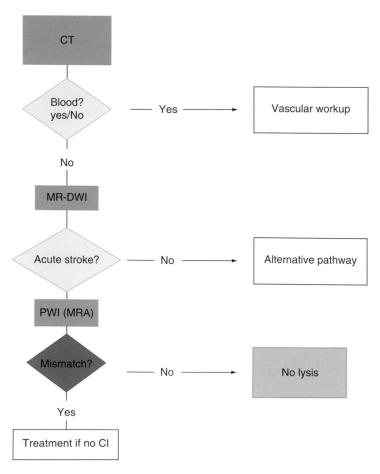

**Fig. 8.5** Exemplary pathway beginning with plain CT which is then supplemented by MR imaging

In this case, imaging can be started with non-contrast enhanced plain computed tomography. This will exclude blood and possibly some of the other stroke mimics. It does not necessitate the injection of contrast. For further assessment, this plain CT can then be supplemented by an MRI examination consisting of diffusion and perfusion weighted imaging. This additional imaging should take no longer than 10 minutes, including patient transfer into the scanner.

Using this pathway has a number of advantages:
1. MRI is highly superior to CT when it comes to detecting any kind of fresh ischemic lesions. This is most pronounced in the posterior circulation. This pathway allows selection of those patients that will profit from the high sensitivity and specificity of stroke imaging that MRI can offer. CT will be able to exclude some of the stroke mimics (hemorrhage) and will also rule out patients with very large areas of already infarcted brain tissue. This reduces the number of patients that will go on to MRI.
2. CT can exclude the presence of metallic objects in the brain (which can often be a contraindication to MR imaging).
3. The MRI team can prepare for the arrival of the stroke patient, which will optimize transfer times between patients.
4. The patient is already in the care of a medical team that can supervise him/ her during the scan.
5. Imaging time is reduced, as now only specific stroke sequences need to be acquired (sequence time <5 minutes).

### 8.1.4  MRI Only Pathway (Fig. 8.6)

MRI is still the most preferred, non-invasive imaging method for the assessment of stroke patients. However, if the MRI pathway causes relevant delay, CT should be preferred.

Magnetic resonance imaging can be limited in severely claustrophobic patients or by implants that are incompatible with MRI, e.g., pacemaker. As stroke patients are often incapable of speech, a body inspection of the patient to screen for scars on the chest (pacemaker) or signs of previous skull trepanation (aneurysm clip) is essential before an MRI can be conducted.

Contraindications for the MRI scan are electronically, magnetically, and mechanically activated implants as well as ferromagnetic or electronically operated active devices (e.g., defibrillators, cardiac pacemakers, metallic splinters in the eye, ferromagnetic intracranial aneurysm clips). Patients with absolute contraindications should not be examined or only with special MRI safety precautions.

> Relative contraindications for MRI scans are cochlear implants and prosthetic heart valves. Most of these are non-magnetic, but if magnetic, they can pose a hazard.

Multiparametric MR imaging can also be used as a first-line screening tool for acute ischemic stroke patients. Total acquisition time ranges from 7 to 15 minutes and can be shortened to sequences that last in the range of seconds. Thus, even in an agitated patient, it will, in most cases, be possible to acquire images that allow the identification of acute ischemic areas.

If you are planning to provide a high-end service, ideally, the accompanying stroke neurologist will have neuro-intensive care experience and will be able to perform slight sedation of the patient, e.g., using Propofol. MRI staff should be familiar with ECG and oxygenation monitoring during MRI scanning.

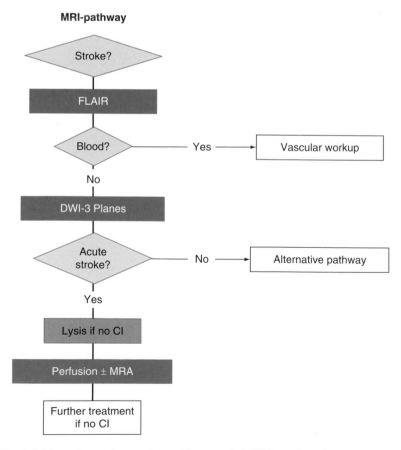

**Fig. 8.6** Exemplary pathway using multiparametric MRI for patient triage

If MRI is used as the first imaging method of choice, this will require FLAIR images that are sensitive to fresh blood. Diffusion-weighted images (DWI images) can detect fresh ischemic lesions (usually in conjunction with ADC maps), and perfusion-weighted images (PWI), as well as MR-angiography (MRA), will give information about the hemodynamic situation in the brain. A possible pathway is shown on Fig. 8.6.

### 8.1.4.1   Order of Sequences Using MR Imaging

The following chart (Fig. 8.7) proposes the order of the sequences when utilizing MRI as the first imaging method of choice. Once an acute stroke is confirmed and contraindications to lysis have been excluded, intravenous thrombolysis can be initiated while the patient is still in the scanner and complementary sequences (MR-angiography, T2* imaging) can be acquired.

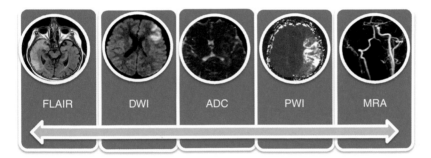

**Fig. 8.7** Order of the sequences when utilizing MRI as the first imaging method of choice in acute ischemic stroke

# Specific Pathways in Special Cases

# 9

Unfortunately, not every stroke is the same, and not every pathway and treatment method will be optimal for the individual patient.

For every 100 patients that are treated with intravenous lysis, three will be harmed and approximately 32 will have at least 1 degree less of disability on the mRS (modified Rankin Scale, see Appendix A.3.1). Even timely administration of lytics does not ensure recanalization. Results from PROACT II showed that vessel recanalization often occurred more than 7 h after stroke onset.

> PROACT II, (Prolyse in Acute Cerebral Thromboembolism II), was a randomized, double-blinded, controlled clinical trial conducted between 1996 and 1998. It compared intra-arterial thrombolysis (using prourokinase) + anticoagulation versus anticoagulation alone for patients with acute ischemic stroke due to distal ICA and proximal MCA occlusion seen on conventional cerebral angiography. Median time to start i.a. thrombolysis was 5.3 hours. It showed that despite an increased frequency of early symptomatic intracranial hemorrhage, treatment with intra-arterial prourokinase within 6 hours of the onset of acute ischemic stroke significantly improved clinical outcome at 90 days. Forty percent of prourokinase patients and 25% of control patients had a mRS of 2 or less ($P=0.04$). Mortality was 25% for the prourokinase group versus 27% for the control group. The recanalization rate was 66% for the prourokinase group versus 18% ($P<0.001$). Symptomatic intracranial hemorrhage occurred in 10% of prourokinase patients and 2% of control patients ($P=0.06$) (Furlan et al. 1999).

In patients with MCA (middle cerebral artery) occlusion, recanalization rates are only 25–30%. For the internal carotid artery results are even worse and do not even reach 10% (Fig. 9.1, Bhatia et al. 2010; del Zoppo et al. 1992; Alexandrov et al. 2004).

I.Q. Grunwald et al., *How to set up an Acute Stroke Service*, DOI 10.1007/978-3-642-21405-9_9, © Springer-Verlag Berlin Heidelberg 2012

**Fig. 9.1** Low
recanalization rate
after intravenous
thrombolysis. *MCA*
middle cerebral
artery, *ICA* internal
carotid artery, *BA*
basilar artery

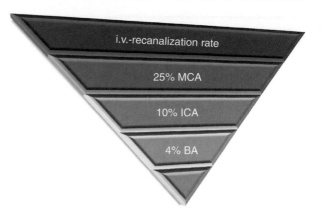

These data suggest that more effective acute recanalization strategies are
needed to further reduce time from vessel occlusion to recanalization and
thus disability and death from stroke.

This next chapter will point out specific patient groups that might profit
from tailored imaging and treatment pathways that can enable alternate
treatment pathways to i.v. lysis.

These groups include:

- Patients with posterior circulation stroke, especially those with an occlusion of the basilar artery
- Patients with occlusion of a major vessel (internal carotid artery, middle
  cerebral artery) that have a low response rate to i.v. lysis
- Patients with wake up stroke where the onset of stroke is unknown

## 9.1    Basilar Artery Thrombosis (Fig. 9.2)

### 9.1.1   Anatomy

The vertebral arteries fuse and form the basilar artery. Together, the vertebral and basilar arteries supply the brainstem and supply the cerebellum
with circumferential branches. The basilar artery ends in a bifurcation forming the two posterior cerebral arteries.

The posterior communicating arteries connect the middle cerebral artery
to the posterior cerebral artery, thus forming part of the circle of Willis.

### 9.1.2   Clinical Features

Some general clinical features of lesions in the vertebrobasilar system
should be noted.

An occlusion of the basilar artery is the location of the greatest concern
in ischemic stroke.

**Fig. 9.2** Basilar
artery occlusion

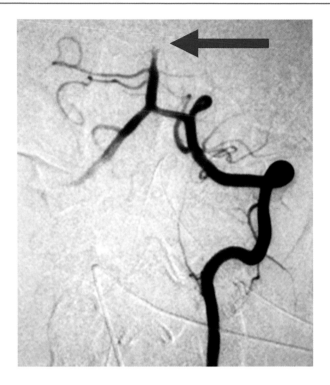

A basilar artery occlusion will result in deficits with complete motor and sensory loss and cranial nerve signs from which patients normally do not recover. The outcome is predominantly fatal, or patients remain comatose. Untreated, a basilar artery occlusion carries a mortality rate of up to 80% (Rumboldt et al. 2009).

In addition, less extensive lesions are often just as neurologically detrimental yet not life-threatening and characteristically result in the feared "locked-in" syndrome. These patients have normal sensation and can see and hear but are unable to move or speak. The patient remains fully alert and orientated but is left with a limit of means of communication that is usually restricted to blinking and upward gaze. Because of the catastrophic outcomes and high fatality rate of patients with a basilar artery thrombosis, aggressive treatment patterns beyond "anterior circulation" time windows are commonly used for these patients.

Results from big endovascular trials (e.g., Pivotal Penumbra) have shown remarkably high recanalization rates, associated with favorable outcomes in a significant percentage of patients that were treated intra-arterially. As basilar artery occlusion is such a potentially devastating disease, these patients should be treated by a team of experts with all therapeutic options, including bridging and mechanical recanalization concepts.

In patients with posterior circulation symptoms and suspected basilar artery occlusion, CTA/CTP should be performed once plain CT imaging has excluded hemorrhage. If no occlusion of the basilar artery is seen but the patient shows a significant mismatch in the posterior circulation territory,

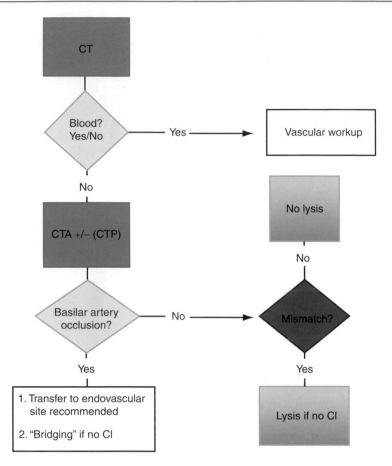

**Fig. 9.3** Suggested pathway for patients with suspected basilar artery occlusion

then occlusion of smaller vessels is likely, and lysis should be considered after exclusion of contraindications. Especially in the posterior circulation, which is difficult to assess in CT, it can be very helpful to perform additional imaging using MRI to better evaluate the extent of ischemic damage. If a basilar artery thrombosis is present, we recommend starting intravenous lysis while arranging immediate transfer to a center that is able to provide additional endovascular treatment, if needed (Fig. 9.3).

## 9.2 Signs of a Major Vessel Occlusion (MCA/ICA)

If a major vessel occlusion is present, this can sometimes already be detected on non-enhanced CT images in the form of a "white" hyperdense artery (Fig. 9.4). In these cases, the chances that intravenous administration will be able to dissolve the clot are low, and early transfer of patients should be considered (Fig. 9.5).

**Fig. 9.4** Hyperdense middle cerebral artery sign

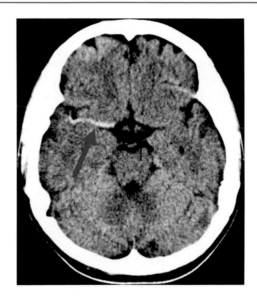

In the middle cerebral artery, i.v. lysis will be successful in about 25%; in the internal carotid artery, recanalization rates are below 10%. In these cases, transfer to an endovascular site can be highly beneficial as recanalization rates using endovascular devices are currently reported as above 90%.

## 9.3    Portable CT Scanners

Portable CT technology allows imaging in every conceivable location. By using portable imaging directly at the emergency site, the hope is to reduce time lost on transport and in hospital management and thus to improve the prognosis of the patient.

Several portable CT scanners are available for clinical imaging. These include the CereTom (NeuroLogica), the Tomoscan (Philips Medical Systems, Best, The Netherlands), the xCAT ENT (Xoran Technologies, Ann Arbor, Michigan), and the OTOscan (NeuroLogica). The Tomoscan was previously used in the Saarland Mobile Stroke Unit (MSU) and consists of a gantry with multisection detectors and a detachable table. It can perform full-body or head scanning. The xCAT ENT is a cone-beam CT scanner that is intended for intraoperative scanning of cranial bones and sinuses. The OTOscan is a multisection CT intended for imaging in ENT (ear, nose, and throat). It is used to assess bone and soft tissue of the head.

9

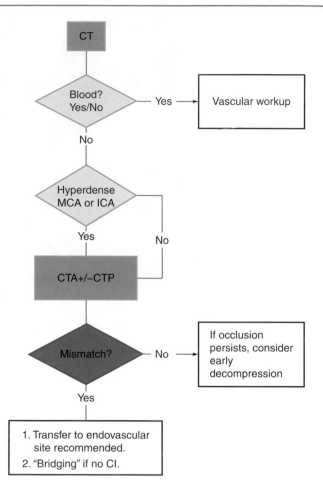

**Fig. 9.5** Pathway for patients with signs of major vessel occlusion. Because of the high failure rate of i.v. rtPA in major vessel occlusion (MVO), we suggest early consideration of endovascular therapy and transfer of these patients to a specialized center

The CereTom 2011, manufactured by NeuroLogica, Corp. is designed specifically for neuroradiologic head imaging and holds an important role in the mobile setting of acute stroke care (Fig. 9.6).

It is an 8-slice small-bore portable CT scanner that delivers high-quality non-contrast enhanced images. The main advantage, however, which singles the CereTom out from other scanners, is that it is the first portable scanner that also provides CT angiography, contrast perfusion, and Xenon perfusion scans in every conceivable patient location (Fig. 9.7).

Due to its size and rapid scan time, this scanner is suitable for a concept such as the MSU (Mobile Stroke Unit, Saarland). In addition, it has an easy to use interface and allows immediate image viewing, which is essential for a rapid

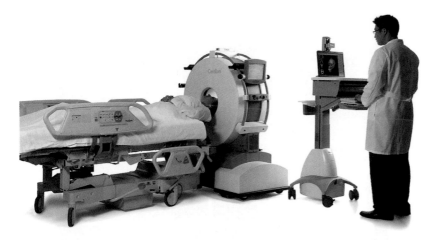

**Fig. 9.6** The CereTom is significantly smaller than a traditional scanner, currently with a height of 153 cm, a length of 134 cm, and a width of 73 cm. Its weight is 362 kg. Eight 1.25-mm-wide detectors provide a 10-mm collimated beam. Typical scanning parameters are 120 kV, 7 mA, and a scanning time of 2 seconds. Reconstructed section thicknesses are 1.25 mm in CT-angiography, 5 mm for head scans, and 10 mm for perfusion imaging. Functionally, this machine can be used to perform CT scanning with and without contrast, CT-angiography, CT-perfusion, and CT-fluoroscopy. CereTom Portable CT Scanner. NeuroLogica Website (Available at http://www.neurologica.com/news-media.html)

decision-making process in patients that present with symptoms of acute stroke. This makes it a valuable tool for any mobile setting of acute stroke care.

## 9.4   DSA with Interventional Treatment as a Primary Choice

In selected cases, interventional treatment can be considered as a first-line treatment in acute ischemic stroke. This should be considered in patients with known contraindication to lysis (e.g., recent operation), in patients with major vessel occlusion, e.g., the internal carotid artery, if lysis failed to reopen the vessel, as well as in patients with marked mismatch in an advanced time setting that would make them ineligible for thrombolysis (Fig. 9.8).

Recently, flat detector (FD)-equipped angiography machines are increasingly used for neuro-angiographic imaging. They can obtain not only high-quality 3D vascular volumes (3D rotational angiography) but also CT-like images (FD-CT) of brain parenchyma that allow detection of intraparenchymal and subarachnoid hemorrhages. Using this technique, images of the brain can be gained without the need to transfer the patient from the angiography suite to the CT. These images provide a low contrast resolution with demonstrated ability for recognition of contrast differences of as little as 10 Houndsfield Units (HU) (Zellerhof et al. 2005).

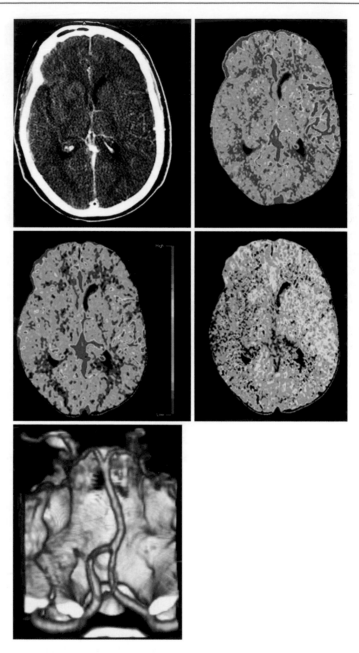

**Fig. 9.7** CereTom: first portable scanner that also provides CT angiography, contrast perfusion, and Xenon perfusion scans

**Fig. 9.8** In selected cases, interventional treatment can be considered as first-line treatment in acute ischemic stroke

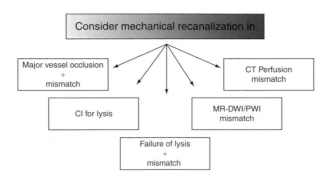

Although contrast resolution is still inferior in comparison to multislice computer tomography, this technique has already been shown to enhance the ability to rapidly recognize and manage common intraprocedural complications (Struffert et al. 2009, 2010).

The ideal setting in which to evaluate a patient with an acute ischemic stroke would be an imaging environment in which assessment of brain parenchyma, vessels, and perfusion as well as treatment could be undertaken in one place, without time-consuming transfer from one imaging modality to another (Fig. 9.9). With the introduction of flat detector (FD) angiography, this has now become a reality in a few selected centers.

Being able to monitor brain perfusion during endovascular procedures can be helpful in the decision-making process as to when to abort revascularization attempts (Struffert 2011).

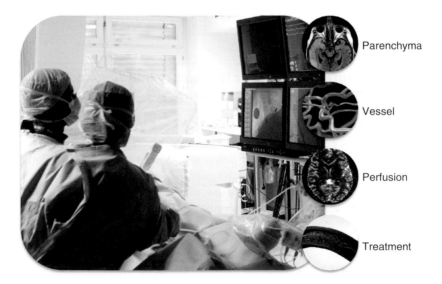

**Fig. 9.9** Stroke assessment including imaging of brain parenchyma, vessels, and perfusion can take place on high-end angiography machines where additional treatment can also be performed

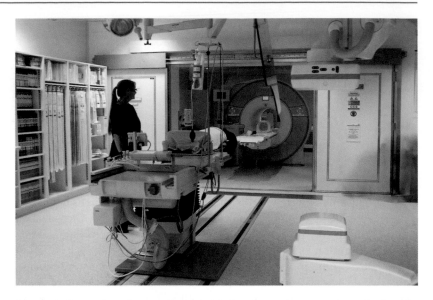

**Fig. 9.10** Integration of magnetic resonance imaging and x-ray angiography into the same suite (Acute Vascular Imaging Centre, Oxford)

Another advantage of FD imaging is the potential to reduce the amount of contrast medium and the dose of radiation that is conventionally needed for patient evaluation. It is possible to obtain both flat detector CT-angiography as well as cerebral blood flow (CBV) from a single acquisition. With conventional computer tomography, two acquisitions and two injections of contrast medium are required to obtain the same data.

## 9.5 Integrated Magnetic Resonance Imaging and X-Ray Angiography

Intraoperative and interventional MRI procedures have motivated continued development of new imaging systems. Fully integrated, intraoperative imaging systems for neurosurgery and neuroradiology are on the market. Some companies now offer an integrated magnetic resonance imaging and biplane angiography system for neurovascular care to provide the clinician with image-guided therapy solutions that best meet the needs of the patient (Fig. 9.10).

With an integrated imaging system, the idea is that after diagnostic scanning using magnetic resonance tomography, image-guided endovascular treatment can commence on the biplane angiography system without additional time delay and without moving the patient from the table.

In selected cases, intraprocedural MR images can also be used with real-time fluoroscopy to assist catheter navigation. Naturally, safety and workflow as well as room controls need to be addressed. Designed for stroke management and neurovascular care, a comprehensive range of interventions can be performed with or without the benefit of MR imaging. Another main advantage is that safe and time-efficient patient transfer between imaging modalities can now be done at any time during the procedure, without moving the patient from the table.

Integration into a fully functional MR imaging room can maximize utilization of the two components of the system. With x-ray angiography and fluoroscopy, the angiography system helps improve visualization.

The ability to visualize intra- and extracranial arteries and to quickly assess the condition of a patient's brain tissue is a major advantage in modern stroke treatment. Using an integrated system, imaging can be done not only before but also during and following interventional neurovascular procedures.

# References

Alexandrov AV, Molina CA, Grotta JC, Garami Z, Ford SR, Alvarez-Sabin J, Montaner J, Saqqur M, Demchuk AM, Moye LA, Hill MD, Wojner AW (2004) Ultrasound-enhanced systemic thrombolysis for acute ischemic stroke. N Engl J Med 351: 2170–2178

Bhatia R, Hill MD, Shobha N, Menon B, Bal S, Kochar P, Watson T, Goyal M, Demchuk AM (2010) Low rates of acute recanalization with intravenous recombinant tissue plasminogen activator in ischemic stroke: real-world experience and a call for action. Stroke 41(10):2254–2258, Epub 2010 Sep 9

CereTom Portable CT Scanner. NeuroLogica Website. Available at: http://www.neurologica.com/news-media.html. Accessed April 2011

del Zoppo GJ, Poeck K, Pessin MS, Wolpert SM, Furlan AJ, Ferbert A, Alberts MJ, Zivin JA, Wechsler L, Busse O et al (1992) Recombinant tissue plasminogen activator in acute thrombotic and embolic stroke. Ann Neurol 32:78–86

Furlan A, Higashida R, Weschler L et al. and PROACT II Investigators (1999) Intra-arterial prourokinase for acute ischemic stroke: the PROACT II study, a randomized controlled trial. JAMA 282:2003–2011

Rumboldt Z, Huda W, All JW (2009) Review of portable CT with assessment of a dedicated head CT scanner. AJNR Am J Neuroradiol 30(9):1630–1636, Epub 2009 Aug 6

Struffert T, Richter G, Engelhorn T et al (2009) Visualisation of intracerebral haemorrhage with flat-detector CT compared to multislice CT: results in 44 cases. Eur Radiol 19:619–625

Struffert T, Deuerling-Zheng Y, Kloska S, Engelhorn T, Strother CM, Kalender WA, Köhrmann M, Schwab S, Doerfler A (2010) Flat detector CT in the evaluation of brain parenchyma, intracranial vasculature, and cerebral blood volume: a pilot study in patients with acute symptoms of cerebral ischemia. AJNR Am J Neuroradiol 31(8):1462–1469, Epub 2010 Apr 8

Struffert T, Deuerling-Zheng Y, Kloska S, Engelhorn T, Boese J, Zellerhoff M, Schwab S, Doerfler A (2011) Cerebral blood volume imaging by flat detector computed tomography in comparison to conventional multislice perfusion CT. Eur Radiol 21(4):882–889, Epub 2010 Sep 21

Zellerhof M, Scholz B, Röhrnschopf E (2005) Low contrast 3D-reconstruction from C-arm data. Progress Biom Opt Imag Proc SPIE 5745:646–655

# Future Concepts in Stroke Treatment

# 10

## 10.1 MSU: The Concept of a Mobile Stroke Unit (Fig. 10.1)

### 10.1.1 MSU: A Mobile Stroke Unit Facilitates Stroke Treatment

The concept of a mobile CT scanner was first introduced by Klaus Fassbender, currently at Saarland University, Germany, and described in "Stroke" in 2003 (Fassbender et al. 2003, Fig. 10.2).

The following pages will explain this novel concept of a "Mobile Stoke Unit" (MSU), a "stroke-ambulance" for pre-hospital stroke treatment that provides all diagnostic tools needed for therapeutic decision taking and treatment directly at the site of the emergency.

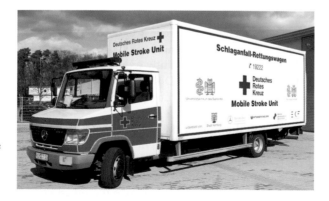

**Fig. 10.1** MSU – Saarland – a Mobile Stroke Unit facilitates stroke treatment

I.Q. Grunwald et al., *How to set up an Acute Stroke Service*,
DOI 10.1007/978-3-642-21405-9_10, © Springer-Verlag Berlin Heidelberg 2012

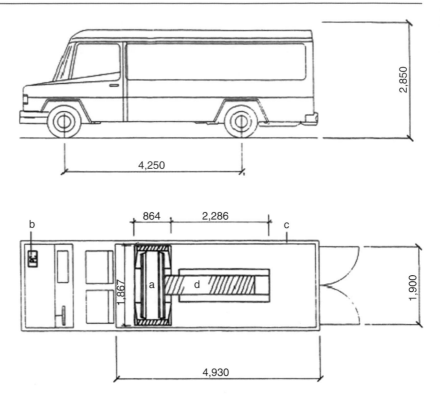

**Fig. 10.2** Design of a "Mobile Stroke Unit" that includes the diagnostic tools necessary for a rapid therapeutic decision for or against thrombolytic therapies: (Dimensions are indicated in millimeters.) (**a**) Integrated small CT, (**b**) operation console, (**c**) isolation against radiation produced by the CT, and (**d**) metal free stretcher as CT table (Fassbender et al. 2003)

## 10.1.2 Rationale

Recanalization of occluded arteries by systemic thrombolysis with recombinant tissue plasminogen activator (rtPA) within 3 hours after onset of ischemic stroke significantly reduces disability and death (The National Institute of Neurological Disorders and Stroke rtPA Stroke Study Group 1995; Adams et al. 2007; European Stroke Organization (ESO) Executive Committee 2008).

Although the time window for i.v. rtPA has now been extended up to 4.5 hours, based on the results of the ECASS III study (Hacke et al. 2008), there is still much that can be done and should be done to salvage the ischemic penumbra and improve the clinical outcome. Despite the potential for thrombolytic therapy to improve the outcomes of patients after ischemic stroke, only 15–40% arrive at the hospital early enough to be eligible for treatment (Katzan et al. 2004; Lichtman et al. 2009; Sandercock et al.

2008). There is general agreement that timely treatment of stroke by rtPA thrombolysis is of crucial relevance for the clinical outcome. However, timely thrombolysis is very difficult to realize in clinical practice since this depends on the very fast onset of diagnostic procedures such as neurological examination, imaging, and laboratory analyses, as well as a timely arrival of the patient in the hospital. Delays here are the major reason why only few eligible patients obtain this often life-saving therapy. Currently it is estimated that only 1.8–3.0% of all ischemic stroke patients in the United States are treated with rtPA (Qureshi et al. 2005; Kleindorfer et al. 2008).

Currently the pre-hospital phase obtains increasing attention, as it is claimed to be responsible for most of the delay in stroke management. This suggests that acute stroke management needs to be reconfigured to allow rapid screening and treatment of stroke patients for the time-limited therapy of acute ischemic stroke. Rapid administration of thrombolytic therapy increases the likelihood of a favorable outcome in ischemic stroke. But quick decision making for the use of recombinant tissue plasminogen activator (rtPA) requires rapid access to strategic clinical data as well as timely exchange of information between the various frontline medical providers and stroke specialist to reduce the "symptom-onset-to-needle times" for a favorable outcome in ischemic stroke.

Treating acute stroke immediately at the site where the patient is found, rather than postponing treatment until hospital arrival, can prevent irreversible damage in vulnerable brain tissue, thereby reducing individual suffering and costs for stroke care for years and decades. This strategy also enables timely planning and preparation of endovascular therapy.

### 10.1.3  MSU: Mobile Stroke Unit

The MSU incorporates multimodal imaging (computer tomography, CT-angiography, CT-perfusion), a point-of-care laboratory, and vast stroke medicine competence represented by a stroke medicine-trained physician, a neuroradiologist, and telemedicine contact to other hospital experts. In short, it combines all that is necessary for ischemic stroke treatment and rational patient triage directly at the site of emergency.

The idea is that by bringing key emergency services directly to the patients' doorstep, thus reducing the symptom to diagnosis time, the mobile stroke unit (MSU) can potentially increase the number of patients that can receive thrombolytic therapy. In addition, with all clinical data already at hand, patients can be individually triaged to further medical treatment upon arrival at the hospital.

In a team effort, the stroke team at Saarland University realized this challenging project in 2008 and started the world's first MSU, which is currently running as part of a randomized trial (clinicaltrials.gov).

Subsequently this concept has been adopted by other centers in Germany and further mobile stroke units are planned internationally. The first clinical results of the MSU were published in 2010 (Walter et al. 2010).

### 10.1.4  MSU: Setup

The MSU is an ambulance (Mercedes-Benz Vario 815D), which apart from the conventional ambulance equipment, incorporates  an accumulator-driven and lead-shielded CT (CereTom, NeuroLogica Corp. California, Fig. 10.3).

This CT is designed specifically for neuroradiological head imaging. It is an 8-slice small-bore portable CT scanner that delivers high quality non-contrast enhanced images and also provides CT angiography, contrast perfusion, and Xenon perfusion scans.

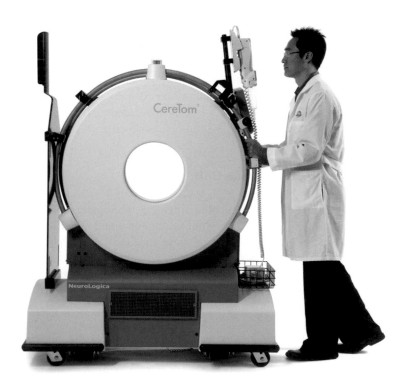

**Fig. 10.3** CereTom, NeuroLogica Corp, California, US

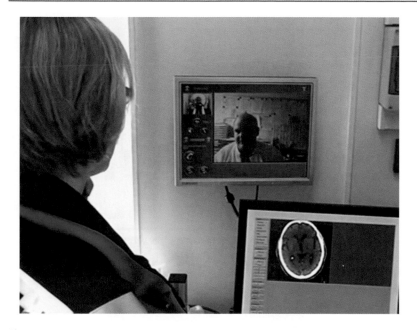

**Fig. 10.4** Telemedicine system

The MSU is also equipped with a telemedicine system (Fig. 10.4) enabling transmission of "digital imaging and communication" data from CT scans or real-time video of clinical examinations of patients via UMTS, i.e., high-speed downlink packet access or alternative network standards to the "picture archiving and communication system" of the hospital.

It is completed with a point-of-care laboratory system (Fig. 10.5). With the latter, platelet count, leukocyte count, erythrocyte count, hemoglobin and hematocrit, international normalized ratio, activated partial thromboplastin time, $\gamma$-glutamyltransferase, p-amylase, and glucose are quantified as requested by current stroke management guidelines (Adams et al. 2007; European Stroke Organization Executive Committee 2008).

The MSU provides on-site clinical expertise in the form of a paramedic, a physician trained in stroke medicine, and a neuroradiologist (Fig. 10.6).

Contrary to current practice, stroke treatment can now be planned and tailored to the specific needs of the patient (ischemic or hemorrhagic stroke) in the pre-hospital phase. Immediate diagnosis of cerebral ischemia and exclusion of thrombolysis contraindications will also allow timely pre-hospital rtPA thrombolysis.

**Fig. 10.5** Point-of-care laboratory

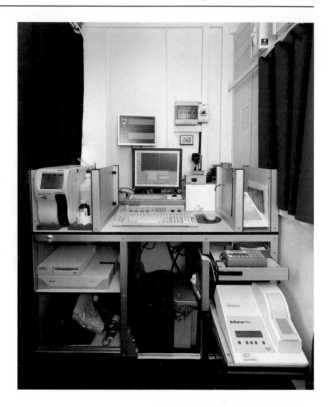

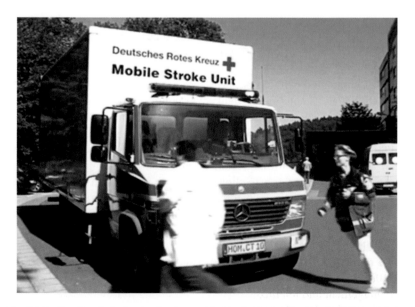

**Fig. 10.6** On-site clinical expertise is provided in the form of a paramedic, a physician trained in stroke medicine, and a neuroradiologist

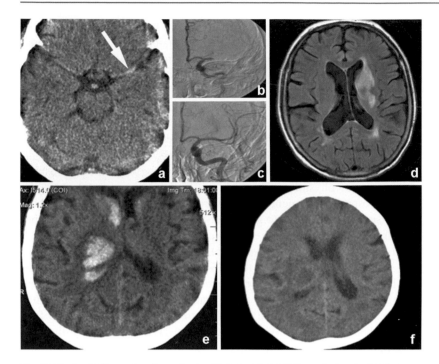

**Fig. 10.7** (**a–d**) Example of a patient with left sided MCA occlusion (**a, b**) that was mechanically recanalized (**c**) FLAIR imaging shows a small, residual infarction. (**e–f**) Example of a patient with hemorrhagic stroke where pre-hospital CT shows intracerebral blood (**e**). CT at 24 hours shows the residual lesion (**f**)

Example of a patient diagnosed in the MSU (Fig. 10.7 a–d). Patient with ischemic stroke: Pre-hospital CT excluded contra-indications for thrombolysis as a pre-condition for initiation of pre-hospital rtPA thrombolysis (Fig. 10a). The "hyperdense middle cerebral artery" sign (*arrow*) suggested a middle cerebral artery occlusion that was later confirmed by digital subtraction angiography (DSA) (Fig. 10b), and it was reopened by intra-arterial recanalization (10c). Magnetic resonance imaging at day seven showed the residual infarction (10d)

Example of patient with hemorrhagic stroke (Fig. 10.7 e–f): Patient with hemorrhagic stroke: Pre-hospital CT scanning allowed immediate diagnosis of intracerebral hemorrhage with ventricular extension (10e), as a pre-condition for pre-hospital differential blood pressure management and telemedicine consultation with hospital experts. CT performed at day 24 shows the residual lesion (10f).

The MSU is not limited to the delivery of pre-hospital thrombolysis. As the name implies, the MSU encompasses all major aspects of pre-hospital stroke medicine such as the pre-hospital initiation of bridging therapy that has recently been shown highly successful in acute stroke treatment (Mazighi et al. 2009).

The MSU concept also allows pre-hospital discussion regarding the need for surgical or other intervention with hospital experts. This can be done via telemedicine, which allows not only the transfer of images but the assessment of the patient as well as video-conferencing.

Using this concept, guideline-adherent and etiology-specific pre-hospital management of physiological variables (i.e., blood pressure) is possible. This pre-hospital assessment will allow transfer to the most appropriate hospital or specialist care unit (e.g., a more distant hospital that can offer specialist services such as a stroke unit, neurosurgery or neuroradiology vs. a closer hospital without those resources).

It was recently shown that the MSU's call-to-therapy-decision times could be reduced to 35 min, with patients demonstrating good clinical outcomes (Walter 2010). These times dramatically break current time limits for stroke management, i.e., the door-to-therapy decision times of 60 minutes defined as a goal by current guidelines (Adams 2007) or the over 60 minutes encountered in daily clinical practice (European Stroke Organization 2009). The considerable time gain resulted not only from reduced times spent in transport or diagnostic work up, but also from increased efficiency in crucial interfaces between paramedics, emergency physicians, neurologists, neuroradiologists, neurosurgeons, or laboratory personnel. In the future, such a MSU can be miniaturized and could include future diagnostic and therapeutic tools (e.g., biomarkers, sono-thrombolysis, neuroprotectives, or hemorrhage treatments), if proven to be relevant (Howells and Donnan 2010).

Though large, randomized multicenter studies are needed to conclusively establish the benefit, the optimal setting (rural vs. urban), the optimal integration in the regional emergency chain (e.g., dispatching the MSU ambulance alone rather than combined with the conventional ambulance in selected cases), and the cost-effectiveness of this MSU concept, the first experience demonstrates that delivery of guideline-adherent and etiology-specific treatment in the pre-hospital phase of stroke is feasible in clinical practice. There are arguments for the assumption that the higher financial investment in the "golden hour" of stroke could offset considerably higher costs over the years and decades of disability caused by suboptimal stroke treatment.

**Fig. 10.8** Stroke pathway using the MSU –
Mobile Stroke Unit. EMS = Emergency
medical service

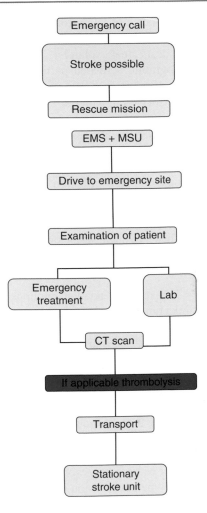

Emergency call

Stroke possible

Rescue mission

EMS + MSU

Drive to emergency site

Examination of patient

Emergency treatment

Lab

CT scan

If applicable thrombolysis

Transport

Stationary stroke unit

### 10.1.5  Stroke Pathway Using the MSU: Mobile Stroke Unit (Fig. 10.8)

## 10.2   New Strategies for Reduction of the Door-to-Needle Times

### 10.2.1  Point-of-Care Laboratory

As we all know time-consuming diagnostic work up is required before administration of i.v. lysis, and implementation of rtPA therapy is difficult to achieve. A major obstacle in hyperacute stroke management is timely performance of laboratory examinations in a centralized hospital laboratory. Current guidelines for thrombolysis recommend that specific laboratory tests (e.g., platelet count, leukocyte count, erythrocyte count, hemoglobin, activated partial thromboplastin time (aPTT), international normalized ratio (INR), γ-glutamyltransferase, p-amylase, and glucose) be performed in patients with suspected stroke in order to identify conditions that mimic stroke or that limit therapeutic options (Adams 2007; ESO 2008; Boehringer 2009).

However, in the "real world setting", results of this time-consuming diagnostic procedure are often not awaited. Indeed, major guidelines even recommend that "although it is desirable to know the results of these tests before giving rtPA, thrombolytic therapy should not be delayed while awaiting the results unless:

1. There is clinical suspicion of a bleeding abnormality or thrombocytopenia.
2. The patient has received heparin or warfarin.
3. Prior use of anticoagulants is not known.

This recommendation might lead to an increased risk of overlooking stroke mimics or patients with contraindications for thrombolysis.

The point-of-care (POC) platform we will now describe consists of mobile laboratory devices that are, in contrast to the centralized hospital laboratory, located directly at the site where stroke patients are admitted to obtain their neurological and imaging examinations. In our case, the point-of-care (POC) laboratory tests are performed by the same personnel who treat the patient, thus potentially reducing interface times and examination times.

Our first results showed that reconfiguration of the entire stroke laboratory analysis to a point-of-care system was feasible and reduced the door-to-therapy-decision times by up to 40 minutes (Walter et al. 2011). Thus, complete transfer of laboratory work up to a POC platform approximately halved the door-to-therapy decision time. Use of a POC platform thus offers possibilities to accelerate stroke management not only directly by reduction of times for transport, analyses or transmission of results but also indirectly, by increased efficiency in interfaces among different health care professionals.

POC-based stroke laboratory analysis may offer a solution to the problem of how to perform necessary laboratory assessments within a critical time frame (Fig. 10.9).

## 10.3   The Acute Vascular Imaging Concept Using Integrated Imaging

Rapid assessment and treatment of stroke is critical. MR imaging and perfusion/diffusion mismatch analysis have been shown to identify areas of salvageable brain tissue in acute stroke and can assist clinicians in quickly determining specific interventional strategies. CT imaging is a sensitive tool to rule out intracranial hemorrhage.

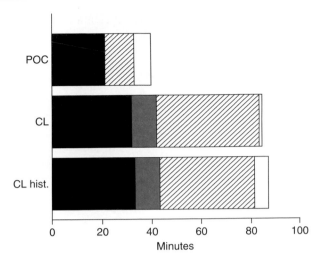

**Fig. 10.9** Comparison of delay of acute stroke management caused by POC-based and centralized laboratory (CL)-based laboratory work up. Moreover, the timing of laboratory management of a historical control group (CL hist.) is presented. The door to therapy-decision time is broken down into the following subintervals: door-to-start of laboratory analysis (*black bars*), until end-of-centrifugation (*gray bars*), until analysis-end and result transmission (*bars with diagonal lines*), and until therapy decision (*white bars*)

### 10.3.1 Flat Detector (FD) Computer Tomography

Modern angiography systems can generate CT-like imaging right on the angiography system. These images are reconstructed from a rotational acquisition, which can also be overlaid with a 3-dimensional image of the vasculature. Thus, soft tissue, the bone, and other body structures can be assessed before, during or after an interventional procedure. Also, high-resolution images of intracranial arteries can be acquired in the interventional x-ray suite. This is based on intravenous injection and is less invasive than a regular intra-arterial contrast injection. By displaying the vessel structure before and after the clot, location of a cerebral occlusion can be visualized.

Especially in critical situations, when the patient's condition may have deteriorated – having access to soft tissue imaging without needing to transport the patient can become important.

### 10.3.2 Integrated Systems

A technology that integrates the operation of a computer tomography or magnetic resonance scanner with an angiography system in one suite has many obvious advantages and can provide the images and information needed to allow personalized treatment decisions and interventions – all in

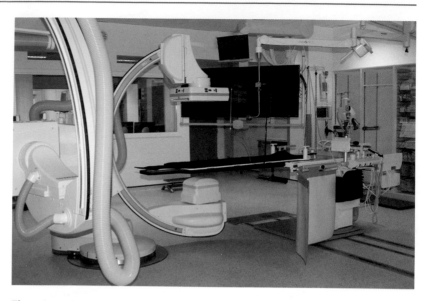

**Fig. 10.10** Integrated imaging system within the Acute Vascular Imaging Centre, University of Oxford, UK

a single integrated system and operating area (Chicoine 2011, Ede 2008, Hushek 2008, Lang 2011).

The concept of the Acute Vascular Imaging Centre in Oxford comprises an interventional suite with biplane x-ray angiography that can be combined with high-field magnetic resonance imaging. This makes it ideally designed for neurovascular care, and stroke management in particular. A three-tesla MRI scanner supplies high-resolution images and critical information. With its high-field MR scanner, the Acute Vascular Imaging Centre provides the ability to promptly identify stroke patients who are likely to benefit from immediate intervention. The integration into a fully functional MR imaging room maximizes utilization of the system (Fig. 10.10).

By using magnetic resonance tomography instead of CT-perfusion techniques to assess the conditions in the brain, the patient is not exposed to ionizing radiation.

The Angio-MRI system MIYABI Siemens, Miyabi being the Japanese word for "elegance", combines the advances of a modern angiography suite with high-end MR imaging technology, thus offering a wide range of advantages for interventional procedures. With this integrated technique, diagnosis of acute ischemic stroke can be immediately followed by interventional treatment and evolution of strokes monitored either by the flat detector (FD) equipped C-arm system itself or by perfusion/diffusion MRI. The resulting reduction in transfer times between the different modalities reduces patient risk and allows a fast double-check of efficacy of the treatment. It also facilitates decision making during the interventional procedure without time consuming preparation for transfer. Especially during interventional recanalization procedures, assessing the amount of potentially salvageable tissue using MRI, can aid in the decision making process of further treatment, thus offering a wide range of advantages for interventional procedures.

The integration of magnetic resonance imaging and x-ray angiography in the same suite for stroke management and neurovascular care is a revolution in modern stroke care. It allows the acquisition of high-quality MR images during and immediately after the procedure, to assess treatment and to determine if further intervention is required. The vast potential of this integrated, high-end technology mirrors the advances provided by endovascular stroke therapy that have currently revolutionized stroke treatment.

Any single, integrated imaging system will streamline workflow and eliminate patient transport between imaging modalities as well as allow evaluation of the efficacy of dedicated therapies (Fig. 10.11).

10

**Fig. 10.11** Example of the Flat Detector Angiographic Computed Tomography (FD-ACT) system "Miyabi" Siemens, Erlangen, Germany that is combined with MR imaging

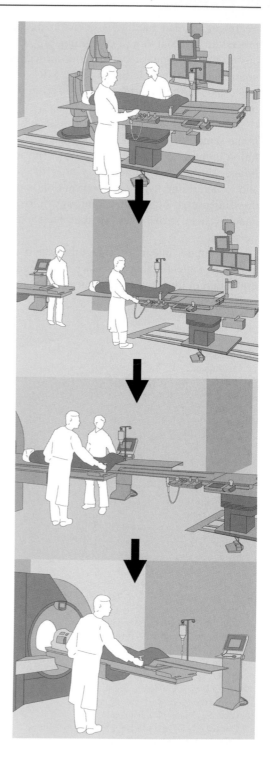

# References

Adams HP Jr, del Zoppo G, Alberts MJ et al (2007) Guidelines for the early management of adults with ischemic stroke: a guideline from the American Heart Association/ American Stroke Association Stroke Council, Clinical Cardiology Council, Cardiovascular Radiology and Intervention Council, and the Atherosclerotic Peripheral Vascular Disease and Quality of Care Outcomes in Research Interdisciplinary Working Groups: the American Academy of Neurology affirms the value of this guideline as an educational tool for neurologists. Circulation 115:e478–e534

Boehringer (2009) Summary of product characteristics last updated on the eMC: 13/08/2009 http://www.medicines.org.uk/emc/document.aspx?documentId=308

Chicoine MR, Lim CC, Evans JA, Singla A, Zipfel GJ, Rich KM, Dowling JL, Leonard JR, Smyth MD, Santiago P, Leuthardt EC, Limbrick DD, Dacey RG (2011) Implementation and preliminary clinical experience with the use of ceiling mounted mobile high field intraoperative magnetic resonance imaging between two operating rooms. Acta Neurochir Suppl 109:97–102

Ede M, Saunders J (2008) Development of IMRISCardio, an integrated, interventional angio-MR imaging suite. EuroIntervention 4(1):154–157

European Stroke Organization (ESO) Executive Committee: Collective Name: ESO Writing Committee (2008) Guidelines for management of ischaemic stroke and transient ischaemic attack 2008. Cerebrovasc Dis 25:457–507 and later revisions

Fassbender K, Walter S, Liu Y, Muehlhauser F, Ragoschke A et al (2003) "Mobile stroke unit" for hyperacute stroke treatment. Stroke 34:e44

Hacke W, Kaste M, Bluhmki E, Brozman M, Dávalos A, Guidetti D, Larrue V, Lees KR, Medeghri Z, Machnig T, Schneider D, von Kummer R, Wahlgren N, Toni D, ECASS Investigators (2008) Thrombolysis with alteplase 3 to 4.5 hours after acute ischemic stroke. N Engl J Med 359(13):1317–1329

Howells DW, Donnan GA (2010) Where will the next generation of stroke treatments come from? PLoS Med 7(3):e1000224, Mobile Stroke Unit PLoS

Hushek SG, Martin AJ, Steckner M, Bosak E, Debbins J, Kucharzyk W (2008) MR systems for MRI-guided interventions. Magn Reson Imaging 27(2):253–266, Review

Katzan IL, Hammer MD, Hixson ED, Furlan AJ, Abou-Chebl A, Nadzam DM (2004) Utilization of intravenous tissue plasminogen activator for acute ischemic stroke. Arch Neurol 61:346–350

Kleindorfer DLC, White G, Curtis T, Brass L, Koroshetz W, Broderick JP (2008) National US estimates of rt-PA use: ICD-9 codes substantially underestimate. Stroke 39:924–928

Lang MJ, Greer AD, Sutherland GR (2011) Intra-operative MRI at 3.0 Tesla: a moveable magnet. Acta Neurochir Suppl 109:151–156

Lichtman JH, Watanabe E, Allen NB, Jones SB, Dostal J, Goldstein LB (2009) Hospital arrival time and intravenous t-PA use in US academic medical centers, 2001–2004. Stroke 40:3845–3850

Mazighi M, Serfaty JM, Labreuche J, Laissy JP, Meseguer E et al (2009) Comparison of intravenous alteplase with a combined intravenous-endovascular approach in patients with stroke and confirmed arterial occlusion (RECANALIZE study): a prospective cohort study. Lancet Neurol 8:802–809

Qureshi AI, Suri MF, Nasar A, He W, Kirmani JF et al (2005) Thrombolysis for ischemic stroke in the United States: data from National Hospital Discharge Survey 1999–2001. Neurosurgery 57:647–654

Sandercock P, Lindley R, Wardlaw J, Dennis M, Lewis S, Venables G, Kobayashi A, Czlonkowska A, Berge E, Slot KB, Murray V, Peeters A, Hankey G, Matz K, Brainin M, Ricci S, Celani MG, Righetti E, Cantisani T, Gubitz G, Phillips S, Arauz A, Prasad K, Correia M, Lyrer P, IST-3 Collaborative Group (2008) Third international stroke trial (IST-3) of thrombolysis for acute ischaemic stroke. Trials 9:37

**10**

The National Institute of Neurological Disorders and Stroke rt-PA Stroke Study Group (1995) Tissue plasminogen activator for acute ischemic stroke. N Engl J Med 333:1581–1587

Walter S et al (2010) Bringing the hospital to the patient: first treatment of stroke patients at the emergency site. PLoS One 5:e13758

Walter S, Kostopoulos P, Haass A, Lesmeister M, Grasu M, Grunwald I, Keller I, Helwig S, Becker C, Geisel J, Bertsch T, Kaffiné S, Leingärtner A, Papanagiotou P, Roth C, Liu Y, Reith W, Fassbender K (2011) Point-of-care laboratory halves door-to-therapy-decision time in acute stroke. Ann Neurol 69(3):581–586. doi:10.1002/ana.22355, Epub 2011 Mar 11

# Strategic/Business Management

# 11

In addition to the clinical aspects of setting up of an acute stroke service, there are the business aspects. It can be useful to appoint a person with business skills for assistance, initially as an adviser. This role may well be outsourced during the first phase of the project. Once the service is established, this role can then be handed to someone who will manage the day-to-day running of the service. Most organizations will have personnel who oversee the business aspects of the organization/units, and one would need to negotiate that service. The cost may be incorporated in the established structure at minor extra cost, or it may require outsourcing.

Once again, this should be established at the start of the business case for any venture so that the costs are incorporated. The earlier this is discussed, the easier the transition and success of the project. If it is identified that there is someone within the current structure, then it needs to be decided if he/she will do the initial business plan and risk management and to what extent he/she is willing and able to take on project management.

Another important decision is who will provide the leadership structure within the service you propose. This decision needs input from the medical director within the hospital, as well as from those service providers either directly or indirectly involved in the stroke chain. While clinical knowledge is critical, even more so is the ability to work alongside a range of other specialists whose input is crucial to the success of the project. Skills such as communication, listening, strategic thinking, networking, and respect for others are vital for the establishment of a multidisciplinary service. Finding someone who is dedicated and focused on establishing a service that will bring the most benefit to the patient and the hospital is essential and many clinicians will have loyalties to their

I.Q. Grunwald et al., *How to set up an Acute Stroke Service*,
DOI 10.1007/978-3-642-21405-9_11, © Springer-Verlag Berlin Heidelberg 2012

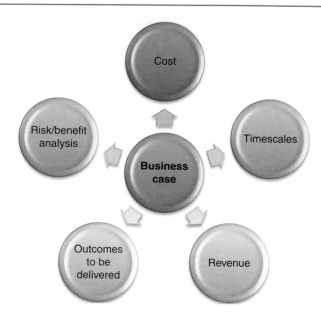

**Fig. 11.1** Development of a business case

own unit/department, but sometimes, hard decisions have to be made in regard to what is best for the service as opposed to what is best for their department/division or themselves.

Once these things have been decided, the business/project manager will undertake to coordinate all the interested parties by setting up a system of communication to keep the appropriate people informed. For some, this is a new drive on their systems that everyone can access; for others, it is via e-mail; for others, it may be newsletters and broadcasts.

One of the early things to develop is a business case. The business case should include the expected costs, timescales, revenue with funding and income, outcomes that need to be delivered as well as a risk/benefit analysis (Fig. 11.1).

The purpose of the business case is to ensure that the project remains justified and that the objectives and benefits being sought can be realized.

If you have stakeholders who have a vested interest in establishing this service, maybe through funding, then they will need to know that the objectives remain desirable, viable, and achievable. The business case will give feedback to stakeholders.

The outline of any business case typically follows the structure of:

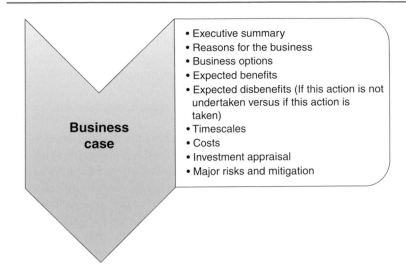

- Executive summary
- Reasons for the business
- Business options
- Expected benefits
- Expected disbenefits (If this action is not undertaken versus if this action is taken)
- Timescales
- Costs
- Investment appraisal
- Major risks and mitigation

Often, when presenting a new business idea, the reason for doing something seems urgent, even essential, and an amazing opportunity to those involved, but frequently, you will need to convince others that this is the case. The business case will give the basis for your presentation to senior management and external stakeholders. They will want to know that your project plan is also aligned with the corporate objectives and strategies.

The business manager will appraise such things as the net benefits, return on any investments, payback period, discounted fee charges, net present value, unseen forecasts and their impact.

Often, the financial aspects are subdivided between the different departments that contribute to building a dedicated stroke team.

VAT or any other type of government tax on goods and services needs to be carefully considered. In some countries, medical equipment is exempt from such taxes. However, it may also mean that you cannot undertake commercial activity within your unit. Once again, this is an expense that requires agreement upon early in the establishment of a Stroke Service that might necessitate additional equipment and machinery. It is tied to the strategic direction of the hospital and impacts on the bottom line should it need to be paid from any income that is made.

Staff costs are the largest ongoing costs to any business. These costs will, in general, be borne by the overarching organization funding the new service. However, some aspects of the service can require additional recruiting of staff. If the running of your Stroke Service requires securing funding for staff, this will be crucial to success.

**11**

As usually, staffing requirements will be determined by the organization's clinical regulations for staff per patient ratio; the issue of staffing is that if they are part of a larger department on a rota, there is a risk that they will not be available to attend to the stroke patient at the unpredictable time when you need them (see risk management).

This will affect operating hours of your service, and you will need to assess the impact on the bottom line.

While being more expensive and not always possible, the ideal situation is to have key dedicated staff working in and overseeing the stroke service. This optimum staffing should include provisions for dedicated nurses and physicians.

Other main costs include the actual equipment as well as staff and usage times, but there are many other costs. Most universities will include these costs within their overhead rate or Full Economic Costing (FEC) model for costing research, but hospitals and other organizations may not have the extra costs included, and they will therefore need to be add-on costs.

In the UK, Universities also receive HEFCE income for the research funds they have raised. This may impact on where funds would be best channeled as these costs may come to the service as extra income. If the Department of Health (UK) is funding the project, it will, by default, send the funding to the hospital, even if it was awarded to someone within the university.

Obtaining a quality certificate by independent authorities, i.e., national stroke societies, is usually linked to constant structural quality measures such as number of examinations, percentage of thrombolysis, use of state of the art diagnostic tools, availability of vascular and neurosurgical services which implies a minimal size of staff per stroke unit bed.

Setting up a functioning Stroke Service is very expensive, and all costs need to be included.

There are many general examples of business plans that can be found on the Internet or through your own organizations. The challenge is to find out which business plan the overarching organization expects. They may have a model that aligns with other activity within the organization.

Gaining data for a business plan when your service has not yet been established can be difficult, and it is advisable to gain costs from other similar services, if you can. Cost and reimbursement of procedures not only varies among countries, but is continuously adapted. This information is, however, crucial to the continued success of the service you are trying to establish and your business/financial manager should be able to give realistic figures on the budget and forecast.

## 11.1   Things to Consider in a Budget

Checklist
1. Who needs to be involved and has information, which will support the preparation of forecasts.
2. Consider how services and other resources will be used and any changes in the competitive environment.

3. Explore variations in activity. For example, is there only an i.v. service available during the night whereas i.a. treatment is possible during daytime?
4. Budget for overheads and other *fixed costs*.
5. Remember to include any *variable costs* and income in the forecast.
6. Identify *non-operational cash flow*, such as taxes or expected changes in funding.
7. The business manager should have experience of payment patterns to forecast the *timing* of all income and expenditure items.
8. The figures need to be presented using a spreadsheet or financial software, commonly called a *cash flow budget*.
9. *Other budgets* could be useful, such as a profit and loss and balance sheet.
10. Your budgets need to contain enough information so you can monitor the *key performance indicators* (*KPIs*) used to manage the business.
11. Identify significant areas of *uncertainty* and prepare separate budgets for different scenarios.
12. *Regularly update* budgets as actual figures become available and circumstances change.

## 11.2 Staffing

Staffing will be the biggest consistent, monetary outlay. It is not just about employing any staff, but it is about employing the "best" people that can work together to build an exceptional team. This is very important, and the success of the unit will depend on decisions made in relation to staff. Some roles are more obvious than others, such as:

- Clinical lead
- First responders (ambulance services)
- Stroke matron or nurse
- Neurologist
- Radiographers
- Neuroradiologist/Interventionalist
- Anesthetist
- Neurosurgeon
- ICU team
- IT expert
- Business manager/operations manager (administrator)

Some of these positions will be easier to fill than others. Writing well-defined job descriptions is important to attract the best quality personnel. After setting the date when you are planning to start your service, you will need to allow 6 months for the recruitment of many of these posts, especially if they are external appointments. Also, candidates might have to set time of notice with their previous employer.

*Once the project is starting, and even when it is running, it is advisable to have* one person as a primary contact. This role is often an operations manager or administrator or it may be the business manager or the nurse manager.

This role is likely to be permanent and can cover any of the following:
- Central point for all correspondence
- Negotiate, write, and manage data: SOPs, services agreements
- Taking minutes at meetings
- Responsible for communications
- Events/marketing management
- Web design and upkeep
- Interact with service providers, maintenance staff, deal with emergencies
- Manage the budget, purchasing, accounts, oversee correct coding of stroke

This role will be the external face for stakeholders, patient's families, others within the organization, and the public. It is important to employ a person who reflects the image you want to establish about your particular hospital service.

Finally, the other most important issue around staffing is who employs them, who pays them, and who decides where they spend their time. As a stroke team is conventionally built of members of different subspecialties (Neuroradiology, Neurology, Neurosurgery, etc.) that constitute an interdisciplinary working unit, your Stroke Service will sit between many clinical departments, all with different priorities and budgets.

There is not one model to fit this issue, and it will depend on your particular organizational structure. Seeking out those who have set up a Stroke Service previously will support your discussion and decision-making. Encouraging your business manager, HR (human resources) manager, and key clinical service managers to talk to their counterparts within other Stroke Services will give your team a good understanding of how others have managed so that you can make the best decision for your hospital within your particular situation.

## 11.3   Who Manages Your Project

You have now established your vision, and it will dawn on you how much work and coordination this will actually require.

Setting up a stroke service is challenging. For instance, it requires coordination of highly specialized professionals – who may have limited experience working together – to achieve a common goal.

However, it is you that is expected to define the right goals, and deliver success, and take accountability for the results.

To manage the set up of a functioning stroke service, that also abides by clinical guidelines and practices, you will need a basic knowledge of the clinical condition "ischemic stroke." Even if you have a clinical background, the success of this complex project requires all of your managerial skills and a keen ability to identify and resolve sensitive organizational and inter-personal issues.

One of the common misconceptions about project management is that it is just scheduling. However, this is not nearly as important as developing a shared understanding of what you want to accomplish or developing a good Work Breakdown Structure (Work Packages) to address all the work that needs to be done.

Although it is common to have clinicians serve as project managers while also requiring that they continue with their clinical work, this can be a prescription for problems. The clinician will inevitably find him/herself torn between managing and clinical duties which means that managing will not get done. You can hope it will take care of itself, but it never does. On a project of this size, it becomes impossible to both work and manage the project because managers are constantly being pulled away from their work by the needs of their clinical teams.

Setting up a functioning, cost effective, and up to date Stroke Service is a challenging job.

It involves:

- Defining the pathways, its features, and its specification and assuring its value both in medical and financial terms.
- Defining the work plan, i.e., how the project will be completed.
- Identifying and creating the project team, the supporting, and empowering team members and uniting them to work towards a common goal.
- Keeping track of everything, identifying problems early, providing solutions, and adapting your plan on the way.
- Managing the dissemination of information and ensuring the continued quality of the service.

In a well-run organization, the teams will treat each other with respect, and be respected within the organization. Also, you will be empowered to achieve the pre-defined objectives and have the authority to make decisions. You will have the time and financial resources and are given the ability to build the team that can and will get the job done.

If your organization does not allow you these tools and the ability to make these decisions, your project can soon become a nightmare.

The clinical chapters in this book can provide you with the knowledge and skills needed to comply with the expectations of a modern Stroke Service.

It is now up to you and your organization to commit to the project's success and do what it takes to establish, run, and maintain an acute Stroke Service.

## 11.4   Project Management Plan

Putting a project in writing helps clarify details and reduces the chances of forgetting something. The following page invites you to take your own notes.

Be aware that often the pressure to produce immediate results makes people skip the planning phase and go straight to the tasks. This will usually create a lot of immediate, uncoordinated activity and increases the likelihood of waste and mistakes.

Inevitably your project will pass through the following four stages (Fig. 11.2):

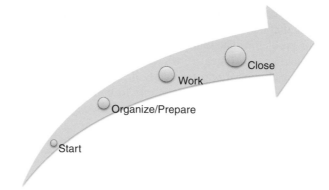

**Fig. 11.2** The four phases of a project

Having asked yourself a series of questions as to the stroke service you want to and can provide, you should now be able to clearly describe the scope of your project and define where it starts and where it ends. For example, "implementing" a new Stroke Service can mean anything from drawing up the concept to purchasing the necessary equipment and software, training people to use it, evaluating the outcome on the patient, and being available for future problems that might occur (Fig. 11.3).

These things should be included in your project management plan:
1. Reasons for the project
2. Description of intended results
3. Constraints
4. Assumptions
5. Resources: personnel, funds, non-personnel resources, equipment, facilities, information
6. Who will play which role?
7. Schedules
8. Risk assessment
9. Work packages
10. Quality assessment

If you have read the previous chapter's points, you will already have some ideas and answers to points 1–5. The following chapters will address specific aspects that need to be considered for points 6–10.

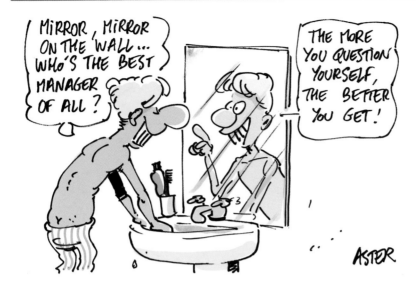

**Fig. 11.3** Ask yourself a series of questions regarding the stroke service you want to provide

# Part II
# Planning

# Establishing Whom and What You Need in the Stroke Pathway

**12**

At this stage, you will have a clear definition of your project and its proposed results. This will help you identify the appropriate team.

The setup and its process will be defined by:
1. Your specific goals (e.g., setting up at 24/7 Stroke Service)
2. Your time schedule
3. Your resources (people, funds, machines, materials, facilities, equipment, knowledge) (Fig. 12.1)

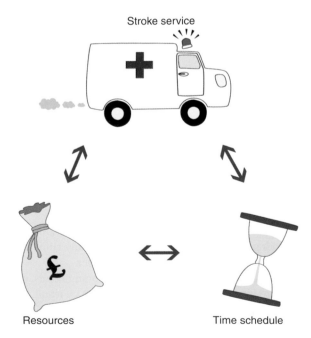

**Fig. 12.1** Image showing the direct relationship between the three main components that define your stroke service

I.Q. Grunwald et al., *How to set up an Acute Stroke Service*,
DOI 10.1007/978-3-642-21405-9_12, © Springer-Verlag Berlin Heidelberg 2012

12

The three most important things that will influence your work are: the quality of service you want to achieve, the preparation time given, and the resulting cost. Obviously you will seek to maximize the quality of your service, e.g., 24/7, while keeping costs at an acceptable, ideally profitable level to your hospital.

However, this just scratches the surface.

## 12.1    Who Are the Key Parties in a Stroke Service?

An essential element is to clearly outline the key parties within the stroke team.

The clinical pathway should be agreed on and developed together with the crucial members of the team, which involves emergency physicians, nurses, the stroke team, laboratory and radiology services, and hospital administration.

You will realize the distinction between "the key parties in a stroke service" and the "key people" that you can ultimately engage in the actual setup process (Fig. 12.2).

Instead of relying on the clinical leads of each department to attend your planning meetings, or to actually restructure and redesign the new aspects of the Stroke Service themselves, it seems a far better approach to select a few individuals who have the aptitude and the desire to be project managers and to let them manage different parts of your work packages.

It is however essential to inform and engage all parties involved in the initial planning meetings to explain reasons for change, possible risks, and benefits involved and to ideally compromise on the pathway you envision.

Be aware that your key partners' professional interests and working relationships are commonly with others in their individual organization, and their boss, who gives them their work assignments and also evaluates their performance.

## 12.2    Meeting Resistance

In setting up a completely new service or even when optimizing the service, be prepared for other people to fight your attempts. In many clinical scenarios, team members have no direct authority over each other.

In addition, conflicts over budget, resources, time commitments, or technical direction may require input from a number of sources. As a result, they cannot be settled with one, unilateral decision.

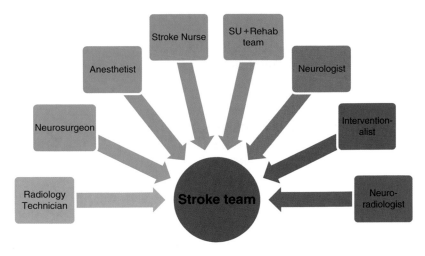

**Fig. 12.2**   The key members of the in-hospital stroke team

As you most likely do not have authority over all the people who will determine the chances for your project's success, get an ally! This should be someone who does have that authority. This ally can help resolve team members' interpersonal conflicts, individual resistance, and busy schedules, and also raise your project's credibility and visibility in the organization.

It can be an endless process encouraging everyone to develop his or her own idea of a Stroke Service. In all likelihood, the individual concepts that will emerge will reflect more the individual's idea of profit, either financially or in recognition, than the common goal. In most cases, it will be up to you to define a clear pathway that finds general support. For this, you need to be crystal clear when stating your project's objectives. The more specific your project objectives are, the greater your chances are of getting them done. Here is some advice:

Put your objectives in writing:
- Be brief when describing each objective. Anything that exceeds half a page will most likely not be read.
- Keep it simple and do not use acronyms.

**12**

When the key stakeholders and parties buy into your objectives, you have the greatest chance that people will work their hardest to achieve them.

If the key parties you previously identified do not support your objectives, work with them to identify their concerns and develop approaches they think can work.

## 12.3   Who Are the Key Parties That Need to be Informed?

In addition, it can be useful to create a list of people that should be informed of the progress.

You will be less likely to overlook people when you consider them department by department or by group, instead of trying to identify everyone from the organization individually.

You can use *the six steps of the Stroke Service* to cover all professions within the acute stroke pathway. It can include those people needed for the project as well as those who are willing to support it.

*Example*:
**People and groups inside your organization**

- Whoever requests the setup of the Stroke Service
- Upper management (Medical Director, Divisional chairs, etc.)
- Project manager, if not yourself
- Affected parties in the stroke pathway
- Team members in the setup process
- Groups that are usually involved
- Groups needed just for this project

*Example*:
**External people and groups that are outside your organization**

- Stroke societies
- Industry and vendors, suppliers, e.g., new software and machinery
- Regulators
- Professional societies
- The public

# Establishing Your Resources (Equipment, Staff, Space)

**13**

Making a detailed list of the resources that are available will not only help identify any missing parts but also be invaluable for calculating a budget.

Resources should be divided into personnel and non-personnel resources. When, for example, technicians are available for the necessary imaging, but the CT scanner is not equipped with CT perfusion or angiography software or likewise the MRI scanner is not equipped with the suitable head coil or software to conduct diffusion-weighted imaging or perfusion scans, you will encounter delays and unanticipated expenditures. Also, your team members may experience frustration that leads to reduction in their commitment.

## 13.1 Determining Non-personnel Resources

As part of the planning, you should develop a resources matrix for the main non-personnel resources you have.

Here is a reminder of the six steps to more easily identify the resources currently available (Fig. 13.1).

**Example of a Non-personnel Resources Matrix for the "Step" Imaging**

|  | 8–18 h | 18–8 h | Week-end | Additional notes |
|---|---|---|---|---|
| CT | √ | √ | √ | |
| CTA/CTP | √ | X | X | |
| MRI | √ | (√) | (√) | Limited service |
| MRA/MRP | √ | X | X | |
| DSA | X | X | X | |
| Doppler | √ | √ | √ | |

I.Q. Grunwald et al., *How to set up an Acute Stroke Service*,
DOI 10.1007/978-3-642-21405-9_13, © Springer-Verlag Berlin Heidelberg 2012

**13**

Your non-personnel resources matrix should display information for every work breakdown structure – step in the stroke pathway.

Take a note of all the valuable resources and expertise you already have in your center.

For example your organizational structure may have an IT department, a business administrator that is a financial wizard. Dr. Merci has expertise in interventional stroke treatment, Dr. Hounsfield is a trained neuroradiologist, Dr. Brain an expert neurologist, and nurse Barthel has taken a course on stroke management. Mr. Smart has taken a course on hospital management; Mr. Stapler is a good organizer....

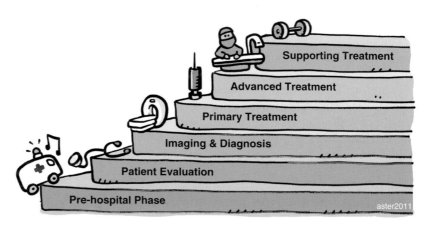

**Fig. 13.1** The six steps of the acute stroke pathway

## 13.2   Determining Personnel Resources

To determine personnel resources, make a list of:

The number of staff, skills, current duties, current level of activity, and times available for each category. These will, among others, include key roles such as neurologist, radiologist, interventionalist, neurosurgeon, anesthetist, laboratory staff, stroke and intensive care unit nurse, and a stroke coordinator. (Fig 13.2):

You have now established your clinical resources.
The same should be done for the managerial sources you have available.

Identify the managerial resources available.

✎ ................................................................................................................

................................................................................................................

The next question you will have to ask yourself is:
What can I change within the constraints of my budget?

✎ ................................................................................................................

................................................................................................................

In Chap. 7, you have developed your own, individual stroke pathway for which you can now estimate the budget. It might then be necessary to modify your concept to comply with your individual resources and the budget assigned.

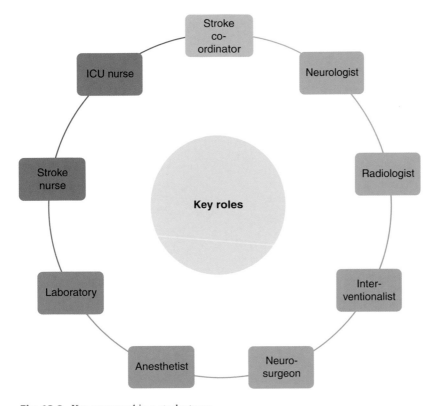

**Fig. 13.2**  Key personnel in a stroke team

# Budget and Time Frame

# 14

The setup of a successful Stroke Service will need appropriate funds. In the current health system, a clear cost/benefit ratio is becoming more and more important.

## 14.1 Benefit-Cost Analysis

A benefit-cost analysis is a comprehensive assessment of all the benefits you anticipate from your project and all the costs to introduce the project, perform it, support the changes resulting from it, and keep it running. It helps you prepare estimates of the resources required to perform the project work. These include: staff morale, labor, capital investment, services, changes in personnel, supplies, materials or maintenance, and service contracts. On the other hand, consider the potential costs of not doing the project.

In a health system with increasingly more limited funds, we are constantly facing the decision on how to get the most return for our investment. Analyzing other already running Stroke Centers in your country regarding their setup, structure and size may also be helpful.

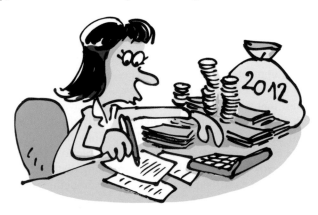

I.Q. Grunwald et al., *How to set up an Acute Stroke Service*,
DOI 10.1007/978-3-642-21405-9_14, © Springer-Verlag Berlin Heidelberg 2012

However, the benefits of a modern Stroke Service with advanced imaging and intervention might well affect the National Health's urgent need, but this could have an adverse effect on your local hospital budget. For example, if the cost for modern stroke devices needs to be covered by your department or hospital, the potential benefit to the patient and a potentially reduced cost in stroke rehabilitation will benefit health insurances but would have no or even a negative impact on your hospital itself.

**Cost-Effectiveness of Thrombolysis**
Cost-effectiveness of thrombolysis was demonstrated in 1998 (Fagen et al. 1998).

Data from the NINDS study was used for this evaluation. rtPA therapy increased the hospital cost by $15,000 per patient, even though it shortened the stay. On the other hand, tPA reduced the cost of nursing home care and rehabilitation. The overall effect was a saving of more than $4 million for every 1,000 patients treated.

It would appear that the willingness and speed to establish modern stroke pathways are directly linked to the amount of government support provided.

Estimating the anticipated costs will show a thorough analysis of all the issues and make your request look professional, helping establish, in the minds of those considering your application, that you are business savvy and likely to run a successful business unit. It will also help you to see whether the necessary funds are sufficient to establish an acute service.

Many hospitals will have business analysis staff that can do scenarios for you, for example, the impact of extending the hours of the unit, the impact of increased superannuation on salaries. These are helpful in determining a business plan showing the immediate plans, 5-year plans and 10-year plans for growth of the business/service.

This cost analysis should be a detailed, time-phased estimate of all resource costs per annum.

When the project is up and running, you can then revise this budget to adapt to changes, e.g., an expansion of the service times.

The service cost is comprised of direct and indirect costs.

The direct costs are the costs for the resources and include the salaries, materials, equipment, and subcontracts (Fig. 14.1).

Indirect costs will include overhead costs.

Ensuring that non-personnel resources are available when needed requires that you specify the times and especially the amount of time that you plan to use them. While it will be impossible to plan the arrival of an acute stroke case in advance, it is however possible to estimate the number of stroke patients that are likely to require immediate inclusion into the stroke pathway. If you then assume that each imaging step will require

**Fig. 14.1** Direct costs

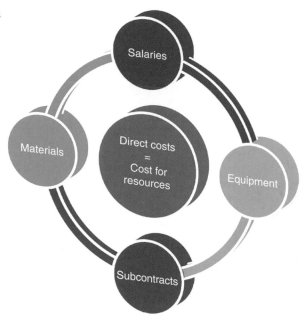

scanning times of 30 min in total, you can then estimate the amount of scanning time per week and year.

Ideally you display this information in separate usage charts for each modality.

### Example of a usage chart

The following figure (Fig. 14.2) of a usage chart illustrates a usage chart that estimates the amount of imaging time per patient at different times and the estimated number of cases per week. In this example, the center is expecting a level of activity of 20 stroke patients a week. Six patients will be imaged via the "MR route," 14 via a "CT route." One of these patients will require additional digital subtraction angiography (DSA) time.

If the average time for imaging is 30 min, the total amount of MR time necessary is 3 h.

Finally, when you have displayed all non-personnel costs for each step of the stroke pathway per week, you can calculate an annual estimation of cost.

**14**

| Activity $n = 20$ | | h | | |
|---|---|---|---|---|
| WBS | | 8–20 h | 20–8 h | Week-end |
| | MR | 6 | 0 | 0 |
| | CT | 10 | 2 | 2 |
| | DSA | 1 | – | – |

**Fig. 14.2** This chart indicates that MR scanning time will be required six times over the week. The expected level of activity per week is 20 patients

## Reference

Fagen SC, Morgenstern LB et al (1998) Cost effectiveness of tissue plasminogen activator for acute ischemic stroke. Neurology 50:883–890

# Risk Assessment and Management

**15**

Risk management includes many aspects, some of which need to be incorporated in the early stages of developing a stroke pathway. As with any project, a Risk Management Strategy should be developed early in the planning process.

The purpose of this strategy is to describe how risk management will be embedded in the daily running of the service as well as the management activities.

Risk management applies from the strategic, operational, program, and project perspectives. For risk management to be effective, the risk first needs to be identified and then assessed – where each risk is ranked in terms of estimated likelihood, impact, and immediacy. This is crucial for understanding the overall level of risk. Identifying appropriate responses to risks, assigning risk owners and the executing, monitoring and controlling of these responses makes risk more controllable.

Local, organizational risk management structures, specialized staff, and documentation will most likely be in place, and SOPs (Standard Operating

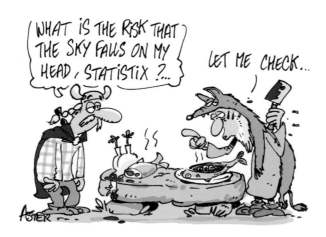

I.Q. Grunwald et al., *How to set up an Acute Stroke Service*,
DOI 10.1007/978-3-642-21405-9_15, © Springer-Verlag Berlin Heidelberg 2012

**Fig. 15.1** Areas of risk

Procedures), policies, protocols and approved practices will need to be incorporated into a risk management strategy.

If you are required to build a unit or just refurbish space, it is a cost-saving measure to involve staff with the authority to approve the clinical space prior to opening.

Areas of risk to consider are infection control, health and safety, and radiation protection (Fig. 15.1).

Once you have decided what type of equipment and space you will need for your Stroke Service, it would be advisable to contact the relevant risk management staff in your organization for their input. Not to do so can be very costly! An example of this was a Stroke Unit that completed its building and had the equipment installed. When the infection control staff came, the unit failed the inspection because it did not meet the required infection control standards. As a result, one of the newly completed rooms required refurbishing to meet the hospital's requirements. This delayed the opening and cost a few hundred thousand dollars on top of the project. At the design stage of the building, the groups mentioned above should have been involved to make sure that the standards, already in place within the hospital, were adhered to in the design.

Due to the type of equipment involved in the stroke pathway, the radiation protection personnel, or their delegates, are important in risk management. Once again, they should be involved early in the process. They will want to ensure that the safety of staff and patients meets the standardized requirements of the organization.

Underpinning the Risk Management Strategy is documentation. Most clinical organizations will already have documentation that can be used, but if this is a new venture, then documentation will need to be developed.

The types of documentation you will need to include:
- Staff *training record*
- Incident *reporting*

- Unit access *management*
- MRI and CT contrast reaction *protocol*
- Entering and documentation of patient data
- Local policies

Note, that the SOPs cover policy documents, reports, management documents, protocols, procedures, forms, and records of important information that will minimize risk. Also, separate SOPs might be required for each area of operation such as MRI or CT.

SOPs need to be kept in an easily accessible place and communicated widely so that everyone knows where to look, should there be any debate on the agreed risk strategies, especially around patient safety.

Involving the correct personnel in the development of the documentation will save time. It is important to be clear who the relevant person(s) are that will approve the Standard Operating Procedures. This part of risk management can be a lengthy process if the documentation is new and should be undertaken early in the process of setting up the Stroke Service.

Patient risk is probably the biggest risk along any stroke pathway. Risk arises from the decision making process.

- When a patient arrives, should he/she go through Accident and Emergency or directly to the imaging center?
- What matrix will be used to assess the patient and what is the best course of action?
- Who makes the decision on a patient's treatment and welfare?
- Whose responsibility is it to ensure the pathway for the patient from arrival to departure?
- What are the risks around transportation of a patient and how will these risks be minimized? Whose responsibility is it to ensure this risk is managed?
- Who reports on imaging findings?: the consultant neuroradiologist, stroke nurse, radiologist, or the person who performs the treatment?

The mitigation of these risks should be agreed upon well in advance of the first patient arriving for treatment and documented in the SOPs.

Another area of risk to consider is the business risk. It would be reasonable to expect a 5-year business plan that shows the operation breaking at least even after 5 years. The risks to this happening can include:

- Non-business people making business decisions,
- Conflicting priorities on the outcomes of the service,
- Conflict between research and clinical use, and
- Conflict of resources.

It is advisable to minimize risk by appointing a business/project manager with financial expertise at the early stages of the project. He/She would also be responsible for overarching documentation where conflict is foreseen.

This documentation will not be necessary for every service but if it is required, it should be considered early in the process.

If there are two different organizations working together such as a university (research) and a hospital (clinical), this type of documentation will be necessary and, once again, needs to be initiated very early on in the process.

In the UK, "insurance risk" pertains to the university undertaking research on clinical patients who are usually the hospital's responsibility. Clinicians are covered by the hospital when they undertake clinical work through professional indemnity insurance cover, but as researchers within the university, they are not covered for clinical work.

"Maintenance risk" pertains to one organization owning the equipment (which is based within the hospital) who can have, often due to lack of resources, a different level of maintenance.

"Staffing risk" pertains to the staff being employed by the hospital within a very busy clinical area where there may be a shortage of resources. If they are being paid by the Stroke Service, but are being managed by a larger clinical department on a rota basis, it will be difficult to ensure that the staff attends acute patients when they arrive at short notice.

Once the Risk Management Strategy has been developed, a Risk Register should be used to capture and maintain information on all of the identified threats and opportunities relating to the operation of a stroke service. In establishing a Risk Register with a database, each risk is allocated a unique identifier as well as details (Fig. 15.2).

In deciding the risk impact, decisions need to be made and recorded. The following is an example of how to record the assessment of risk impact.

| Probability | |
| --- | --- |
| 0.9 | Very high 71–100% |
| 0.7 | High 51–70% |
| 0.5 | Medium 31–50% |
| 0.3 | Low 11–30% |
| 0.1 | Very low up to 10% |
| 0 | Risk identified but agreed no risk |

The Risk Registry can be managed by someone with administrative duties within the organization. A key identifier of excellent organization is having excellent communication, and this will ensure that risk is well managed.

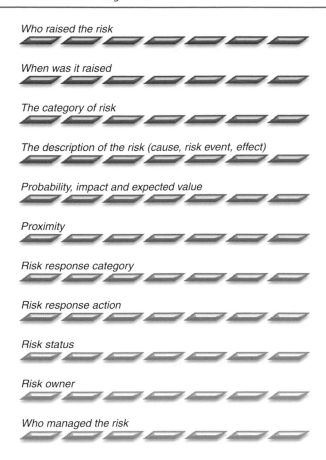

Who raised the risk

When was it raised

The category of risk

The description of the risk (cause, risk event, effect)

Probability, impact and expected value

Proximity

Risk response category

Risk response action

Risk status

Risk owner

Who managed the risk

**Fig. 15.2** Risk Register

# The Team

**16**

## 16.1 Setting Up a Project Team

If you are the project manager, you are responsible for all aspects of the project.

Being responsible does not mean you have to do the whole project yourself, but you do have to see that every activity is completed satisfactorily.

You will not be able to achieve such a complex project on your own, but you will need the support of other team members. For example, you will rely on team members with clinical, technical, financial, or managerial expertise.

It is your job to bring these people and their expertise together to meet the challenges in the project effectively and efficiently.

In general, any person that supports your efforts to set up an acute stroke service should be involved. The only question that needs to be answered is "when" and "how."

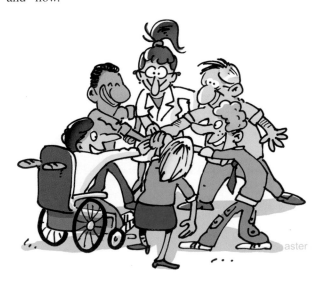

I.Q. Grunwald et al., *How to set up an Acute Stroke Service*,
DOI 10.1007/978-3-642-21405-9_16, © Springer-Verlag Berlin Heidelberg 2012

You have already identified the stake holders of the project, namely, those people that are affected by the success or failure of your efforts.

Now, the team members will be defined. These are all the members of the team that the project manager "directs."

Your project's success rests on your ability to enlist the help of appropriately qualified people to perform your project's work.

Whether you can put the team members together yourself, or are assigned an "imposed team," your first step is to decide which activities you will need to perform and to determine the skills and knowledge people must have to perform them.

You then need to identify those people who are appropriately qualified to address your project's requirements.

Discuss with each team member his or her skills, knowledge, and level of interest in a stroke service.

Other skills you might want to assess are the ability to listen and to express themselves clearly as well as their flexibility.

The next step is to assign each member of the team a task most suitable to him or her to lead work groups that will address the specific aspects that need to be organized on the stroke care pathway. That individual team member is then responsible for delivering the required result on time.

Other people that are not directly part of the team but that will help you accomplish your goals are groups such as human resources, information services, legal services, procurement or contracting, finance, health and safety, and security (Fig. 16.1).

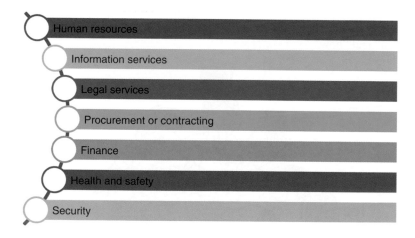

**Fig. 16.1** Group members to involve

## 16.2   Defining Team Members' Roles and Responsibilities

After you have identified the main tasks (work packages) and established the key members of your team, it is time to list them and define each team member's roles and responsibilities. Examples for work packages in the setting up of a stroke service are given in Chap. 17.

To get every work group started, it is important to clarify why addressing this problem is vital for the project. Sharing the available clinical "level of evidence" with the group and explaining the benefit of a functioning stroke service to the individual and also to society can strengthen motivation even more.

# Part III

# Getting Started

# Work Packages

Your entire project can be divided into sub-components. These can again be subdivided into the next level of components. You can continue to subdivide all the components you create in the same manner until you reach a point at which you think the components you defined are sufficiently detailed for planning and management purposes. This lowest-level component in a particular work breakdown structure is called *work package*.

Creating work packages helps remember all the important pieces of work and facilitates accurately estimating the time and resources required to perform that work. The greater the detail in which you decompose a project, the less likely you are to overlook anything significant.

Quickly remind yourself of the three phases in stroke treatment:
*the pre-hospital*,
*the emergency*,
the *post-treatment phase*.

Remind yourself of the components that currently characterize the Stroke Service within your hospital.

Which phases in the stroke treatment pathway have you sorted?

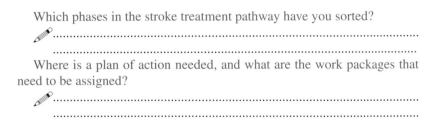

Where is a plan of action needed, and what are the work packages that need to be assigned?

I.Q. Grunwald et al., *How to set up an Acute Stroke Service*,
DOI 10.1007/978-3-642-21405-9_17, © Springer-Verlag Berlin Heidelberg 2012

**17**

| | Yes | No | ? | Plan of action/WP |
|---|---|---|---|---|
| Patient and family will recognize stroke symptoms | | | | |
| Stroke medical contact is available and known, e.g., 112; 999 | | | | |
| Dispatch of the appropriate pre-hospital care provider | | | | |
| Pre-hospital evaluation and identification of stroke correct | | | | |
| Pre-hospital pre-defined choice of appropriate hospital specified | | | | |
| Pre-hospital notification of stroke team | | | | |
| Pre-hospital notification of pending arrival | | | | |
| Emergency setting available | | | | |
| Stroke team established | | | | |
| Emergency work up organized | | | | |
| Evaluation of the patient and initial management defined | | | | |
| Imaging pathway established | | | | |
| Competent interpretation of image results | | | | |
| Assignment to treatment pathway organized | | | | |
| Treatment according to pathway | | | | |
| Disposition of patient to appropriate unit (ICU, stroke unit) | | | | |
| Stroke adapted supervision of patient on ward | | | | |
| Additional medical care organized | | | | |
| Decompressive surgery is available | | | | |
| Rehabilitation organized | | | | |

# Work Groups

# 18

## 18.1  Pre-hospital Phase

### Example 1: Public Awareness and Emergency Services

Consider creating a work group to address public awareness. The people in this work group should include stroke nurses, voluntary stroke organizations, as well as paramedics, media, and local GPs.

You should provide the group with the following background information:

### Background Information
Acute stroke is one of the leading factors of morbidity and mortality worldwide. In industrialized countries, after cardiovascular disease, stroke represents either the second or third most common cause of death.

There is level I evidence that stroke patients should be treated in Stroke Units. Therefore, suspected stroke victims should immediately be transported to the nearest Medical Center with a Stroke Unit or to an organized acute stroke care service. There is level III evidence that once stroke is suspected, patients should call the Emergency Medical Service (EMS).

Now identify the problem at hand.

### Current Problems
1. Patients and relatives often do not recognize the symptoms of stroke and do not realize that seeking treatment is urgent.
2. General practitioners or staff do not recognize described symptoms as stroke and do not notify the emergency chain.
3. Incorrect diagnoses by the paramedical service.

I.Q. Grunwald et al., *How to set up an Acute Stroke Service*,
DOI 10.1007/978-3-642-21405-9_18, © Springer-Verlag Berlin Heidelberg 2012

**18**

These facts clearly emphasize the need for continuous education. When planning a stroke service, general practitioners and paramedical services should be informed and supplied with structured leaflets on stroke symptoms and the existing emergency chain.

### Work Plan and Solutions

This work group should come up with the most efficient ways to reach patients at risk of stroke and their families, large employers, and family physicians.

Be aware that inaccurate initial diagnosis also by professional groups presents a major problem.

Ambulance dispatchers' and paramedics' assessment will have a crucial impact on the patients' pathway. Results can be significantly improved by adequate training.

## Example 2: Education of Pre-hospital Medical Personnel

### Background Information

Physicians and the medical personnel involved in transportation and initial assessment of the patient must be trained and should be able to cope with the early complications after stroke. The medical personnel also needs to be trained in recognizing symptoms and signs of acute stroke and applying stroke scales such as the NIHSS scale. Different aspects of training include the conduct of medical examination, presence of focal weakness, and the concept of 'time is brain'.

### Current Problems

Physicians contacted by the patient or their relatives are not familiar with the local stroke chain and sometimes fail to dispatch the patient to an appropriate center.

### Work Plan and Solutions

A possible solution this work group could come up with is:

### Advice for General Practitioners

The doctor who receives the call should, if a stroke is suspected, recommend/arrange for emergency transportation, preferably through the EMS system, to the nearest emergency room of a hospital providing organized acute stroke care. The relevant contact numbers should be sent to all local medical providers who should then inform their staff, especially at reception.

## 18.2    Acute Phase

### Example 3: Clinical Pathway of the Patient
### in the Hospital

**Current Problems**
Once arrived in the hospital setting, time is again of the essence. Delays caused by transportation within the hospital, lack of pertinent and immediate diagnostic, delayed laboratory and imaging work will severely compromise the patient's clinical outcome.

**Work Plan and Solutions**
A standard hospital routine protocol assigning multidisciplinary staff in the emergency setting and their availability should be established which could include EMS and emergency department staff and their immediate communication with neurologists, neuroradiologists, anesthetist, neurosurgeons, laboratories, and cardiologists, taking into account the emergency situation.

In particular, this work group should:
1. Evaluate current in-hospital pathways and the time delays caused by each step
2. Determine the best strategic step for the patient to arrive, e.g., emergency care unit or CT scanner
3. Review existing guidelines to ensure compliance, e.g., ESO guidelines of 2008 and later revisions
4. Include an estimated cost of such improvements

The strategic admission assessment should be clearly attributed to the relevant staff members, i.e., recording of stroke symptoms, precise or estimated time of stroke onset, conditions under which the stroke occurred, neurological and functional status, dispatching of blood work.

### Example 4: Imaging Requirements

**Current Problems**
1. Unnecessary delays in performing immediate intracranial imaging of the acute stroke patient, tailored to the specific needs.
2. Delays in imaging assessment and reporting
3. Uncertainties about location and availability of the imaging facilities (e.g., operating hours)

## Work Plan and Solutions

This group is part of the crucial in-hospital arrival pathway. Imaging should be part of the routine protocol covering the patient's arrival phase in terms of diagnostic.

First, the existing imaging resources and their availability and staffing should be identified; if these need to be completed, proposals with relevant cost estimates should be made. Also, in case of unavailable parts of the imaging facilities, subcontracting could be considered by taking into account the emergency situation.

The group should work out the most efficient way to start the patient's diagnostic imaging after neurological examination. This involves organization of the different imaging phases in terms of material, staff, and the continuous monitoring of the patient. Smooth transition from the first diagnostic CT to subsequent imaging, e.g., digital angiography for intervention, should be ensured, and their locations and contact points clearly be identified.

## Example 5: Choice of Treatments

### Current Problems

There is a multitude of acute stroke treatments available which range from i.v. lysis alone, i.a. lysis alone, i.v./i.a. lyses combined (bridging) to a growing number of mechanical endovascular treatment options.

### Work Plan and Solutions

Initial i.v. lysis or combined i.v./i.a. lysis (the bridging therapy) is the standard approach for patients within the 4.5 h window after stroke symptoms onset, if no contraindications exist (cf. Chap. 1).

Being able to administer i.v. lysis, when indicated, is the minimum requirement when setting up a stroke service.

The work group should come up with an assessment of the current facilities and expertise within the center (e.g., stroke trained physicians, neurologists, interventional service). It should include an estimated cost of further training for staff, reimbursement of stroke devices, and therapies.

It should also take into consideration that in case intravenous treatment fails to recanalize, mechanical interventions and therapies are available, which might require early transfer of the patient to a tertiary care center. The work group needs to identify approved procedures, interventions, and therapies in acute stroke care and to assess each according to effect of action, level of scientific evidence, and cost-effectiveness. Treatments under investigation should also be considered.

## Example 6: Documentation

### Current Problems
1. Losing oversight of your project
2. Difficulty in identifying situations that may comprise your project

### Work Plan and Solutions
To support the tracking, controlling, and replanning of activities, proper documentation is vital. After preparation of the different work packages, the group should gather all essential information about the different work package components and keep it in a file that is available to all project team members. At a minimum, this file contains information about:
– Title and task description of the work group
– Included activities that must be performed to realize this work
– Scheduled mile stones
– The quality requirements for this sub-project and the required resources, which include people, funding, equipment, facilities, information, and materials

## 18.3   Post Treatment Phase

## Example 7: Patient Transfer After Intervention

### Current Problems
Where to transfer the patient after treatment and intervention?

General stroke care includes a number of factors such as blood pressure and glucose control and nutritional support.

The Stroke Unit Trialists showed an 18% relative reduction in mortality, reduction in death or dependence, and a reduction in death or need of institutional care when patients were treated in a stroke unit, in comparison with a general medical ward (level I evidence).

## Work Plan and Solutions

This work group should evaluate current availability of intensive care beds either within ICU or a stroke unit under consideration of available nursing staff. Patients, especially those with a basilar artery occlusion, might necessitate prolonged ventilation, and often the arterial access line will have to remain for a longer period.

If no dedicated beds are available, the estimated cost of establishing special stroke beds should be calculated.

One solution might be that a dedicated stroke bed is reserved in an interdisciplinary ICU.

If not available, transfer pathways to a suitable unit need to be arranged.

## Example 8: Interventional Management of the Patient

### Current Problems

Interventional management of a stroke patient requires close collaboration with the interventionalist, neurologist (stroke physician), as well as the anesthetist.

### Work Plan and Solutions

This work group should set up a chain that ideally allows stroke to be categorized as a number one emergency, similar to a cesarean. The additional cost for this service should be calculated.

## Example 9: Risk Assessment

### Current Problems

Lack of coordination during the imminent peri- and postoperative phase

### Work Plan and Solutions

The group should identify the actual management of the postoperative phase and define a comprehensive list of follow-up monitoring taking into account the interdisciplinary aspect and the individual risk factors of the patient. Pathologies known to contribute to the occurrence of stroke-like cardiac diseases (in particular atrial fibrillation), cardiovascular problems, diabetes, hypertension, hyperlipidemia should be taken into account by the physicians and nursing staff in charge of these pathologies.

## Example 10: Neurosurgical Management

### Current Problems
Lack of integration of neurosurgeons into the actual stroke team, thus delaying decompressive surgery when needed.

### Work Plan and Solutions
The group should identify the availability and location of neurosurgery which should be integrated into the stroke chain. They can then be on standby in case of complications during treatment or post-operatively.

A predefined member of the neurosurgical team should be identified and informed in advance of a possible candidate for decompressive surgery so that preparations can be done in time and not only when symptoms occur.

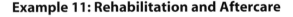

## Example 11: Rehabilitation and Aftercare

### Current Problems
1. Lack of awareness of the importance of early rehabilitative measurements
2. Lack of physiotherapy services
3. Lack of coordination of future care and further medical treatment
4. Lack of information to the patient on supporting measures and help groups
5. Loss of the patient to follow-up

### Work Plan and Solutions
The group should research how patients are routinely discharged and what the patients' options are. The next step should be for the group to organize the coordination after discharge by a dedicated team with either another hospital, a nursing home, or the patient's actual residence in order to update his/her health condition in the hospital file which should be made available to the different hospital departments.

A consensus on general rehabilitation principles should be found, based on available guidelines, with the aim to prevent future complications.

Ideally, a social worker can assist the patient and his family with the numerous formalities involved.

Aftercare should include psychological support.

# Part IV
# Evaluation

# Monitoring

# 19

## 19.1 Project Performance

Monitor your project's performance regularly. This involves monitoring where you stand in setting up the stroke pathway as well as monitoring the effectiveness of the service. You may choose to monitor selected project activities on a daily basis.

Intermittently reaffirm with team members their project and service responsibilities and continued commitments.

Make sure everyone undertakes the activities and provides the service they agreed on and that schedules and pathways are kept.

Also monitor the amount of non-personnel resources used as well as expenditures and income of the activity.

These figures should be collected and, at the end of each evaluation period, compared to the business plan. If it deviates, reasons can then be determined.

## 19.2 Times and Outcomes

To get an overview of any current time delays, it is advised to monitor the times between each step of the stroke pathway. These include the times elapsed between patient arrival in the emergency department until performance of either a computer tomography or MR-tomography, times until the scan is reported, time elapsed between arrival in hospital and a decision on treatment is made, then, finally, the times until treatment is started and the time it takes for a patient to actually get decompressive surgery if he develops a significant brain edema.

I.Q. Grunwald et al., *How to set up an Acute Stroke Service*,
DOI 10.1007/978-3-642-21405-9_19, © Springer-Verlag Berlin Heidelberg 2012

**19**

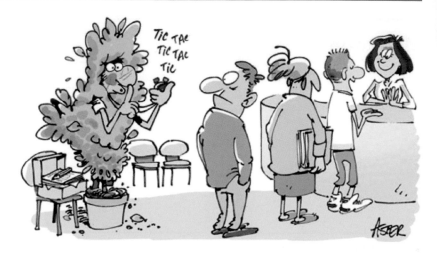

In order to compare and communicate not only the severity of stroke but also the outcome, a common language is needed. From the beginning, it is advised to use and train staff on an established stroke scale rather than defining individual grading systems.

The National Institutes of Health Stroke Scale (NIHSS) score has been extensively studied in clinical trials. Physicians and nurses caring for patients with stroke can be certified in the use of the NIHSS by the American Stroke Association or the National Stroke Association on their respective websites. In addition, training materials can be obtained from the National Institute of Neurological Disorders and Stroke (NINDS) website.

Common types of outcome scales are the Barthel Index, which assesses activities of self-care and mobility, the modified Rankin scale (mRS), which assesses functional independence, and a stroke specific scale, which assesses quality of life. Most acute clinical trials on stroke use the modified Rankin Scale (mRS) at 90 days as a primary outcome measure.

You should estimate the average time between each clinical step and see if there is room for improvement.

Obviously, some parts will be out of your control to change, whereas other areas might benefit from restructure.

The aim of this exercise, tedious as it may be, is not only part of quality control but can nicely illustrate where delays occur in clinical evaluation of stroke patients and in their imaging and image interpretation as well as their subsequent treatment.

# Marketing

# 20

## 20.1 Dissemination

Marketing of the Stroke Service is also critical for the success of the unit. Various options are available but the importance of the web cannot be underestimated in advertising what the unit offers in the way of services. If possible, the web site should be alive when the new Stroke Service opens.

It is not only the external stakeholders who need to be made aware of your Stroke Service and the newly established pathways for patients. Marketing also needs to include:

- Internal staff: admissions, nurses, and porters
- External staff: ambulance drivers
- Patients and their families
- External stakeholders: funders, volunteers, and collaborators

Informing others within your organization is important so that everyone is aware of your existence and especially of pathways that have been agreed for stroke patients once they enter the hospital. Flow charts are a particularly good way of disseminating information and once again the need for excellent communication is required. Holding "open days" and talks will raise the profile of the unit, both internally and externally. Organizations attached to health will often be very interested in supporting new units and should be approached.

Some units will not be required to fundraise while others may need to do some. Once again, Stroke Societies and other health related organizations often have volunteers who are more than willing to help out with fundraising events and eager to lift the profile of your service. If your organization has an events/media coordinator, it is worth contacting him/her in order to support your venture. One would expect this person to be involved a month or two before the establishment of the new service, so that he/she has time to work on marketing material and disseminate the information. If your

I.Q. Grunwald et al., *How to set up an Acute Stroke Service*,
DOI 10.1007/978-3-642-21405-9_20, © Springer-Verlag Berlin Heidelberg 2012

**20**

organization does not have such a person, this may be another position that you consider on a short-term contract for a few months.

In collaboration with the partners involved in the project, other ways of public recognition or revenue streams should be explored. One such idea is the participation in validated trials and registries.

The Way Forward: (things to consider)

Translational research is the way forward; Government and organizations are willing to fund research that is collaborative in nature. Therefore, from a revenue perspective, all avenues in this regard should be explored. Once again the business manager can do much of the groundwork in exploring the possibilities to present to those involved in research and clinical work. The collection of data and publications from existing Stroke Services as well as your own should be analyzed to put your unit at the cutting edge of input into government health strategies.

There will always be core business within a Stroke Service. An understanding of how your service can grow and expand makes good business sense. Collaborations with those services, nationally and internationally, can also improve the work you are doing. If the impact on the economy through an organized Stroke Service is correct, then many countries will be interested in establishing Stroke Services and units that cater to the needs of an acute stroke victim. At the moment EU support is available in particular to those interested in clinical work that will add economic value to the nation. Funding also covers collaborations with other European countries to improve their services.

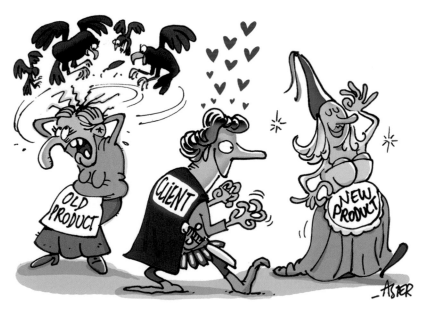

## 20.2   Redefining Your Goals (e.g., Expand Service)

It is important to constantly review the entire process for potential improvement not only regarding image protocols, but also time and effectiveness. Plan to assess the performance of your Stroke Service monthly to promptly identify any unexpected obstacles or performance problems. Reducing the time needed for diagnosis will directly affect morbidity and mortality.

# Closing Remarks

**21**

Stroke is a medical and often also a surgical emergency. Successful care of the acute stroke patient begins with the recognition by both the public and the health professional that stroke is an emergency. The successful care of the acute stroke victim will depend on recognition of symptoms, instant use of the emergency medical system, rapid and accurate diagnosis, and treatment at the hospital as well as adequate aftercare. Establishing a robust Stroke Service remains one of the most challenging, but also rewarding, tasks in the public health sector.

The authors hope that this book will provide insight into the current treatment options and pathways available for stroke management to help you choose the course of action that best suits your needs. After having read this book, we hope you are now full of new desires to take control of your clinical environment and take a lead in modern stroke treatment. You will experience that there is a big difference between knowing what to do and actually doing it. Dealing with the individual strength and the forces that threaten to prevent you from reaching your goals will require all of your interpersonal skills.

As your current service develops and adapts to more imminent needs, we hope you will repeatedly refer to this book and regard it as a source of information that has more to share than the simple knowledge of stroke management, but rather as a book that you can use to adapt to your individual changing needs.

I.Q. Grunwald et al., *How to set up an Acute Stroke Service*,
DOI 10.1007/978-3-642-21405-9_21, © Springer-Verlag Berlin Heidelberg 2012

# Appendix: Tables

**Table A.1** TIMI Grade Flow

| Score | TIMI score/classification of blood flow |
|---|---|
| 0 | TIMI 0 – No perfusion. |
| 1 | TIMI I – Penetration without perfusion. Penetration past initial occlusion but no distal branch filling. |
| 2 | TIMI II – Partial perfusion of the artery with incomplete or slow distal branch filling. |
| 3 | TIMI III – Complete perfusion of the artery. |

**Table A.2** Modified Thrombolysis in Cerebral Infarction (TICI) Perfusion Categories[**]

| Score | TICI perfusion categories |
|---|---|
| Grade 0: | *No perfusion.* No antegrade flow beyond the point of occlusion. |
| Grade 1: | *Penetration with minimal perfusion.* The contrast material passes beyond the area of obstruction but fails to opacify the entire cerebral bed distal to the obstruction for the duration of the angiographic run. |
| Grade 2: | *Partial perfusion.* The contrast material passes beyond the obstruction and opacifies the arterial bed distal to the obstruction. However, the rate of entry of contrast into the vessel distal to the obstruction and/or its rate of clearance from the distal bed are perceptibly slower than its entry into and/or clearance from comparable areas not perfused by the previously occluded vessel, e.g., the opposite cerebral artery or the arterial bed proximal to the obstruction. |
| Grade 2a: | *Partial filling* with <50% of the entire vascular territory is visualized. |
| Grade 2b: | *Partial filling* with ≥50% of the entire vascular territory is visualized. If complete filling of all of the expected vascular territory is visualized, the filling is slower than normal. |
| Grade 3: | *Complete perfusion.* Antegrade flow into the bed distal to the obstruction occurs as promptly as into the obstruction *and* clearance of contrast material from the involved bed is as rapid as from an uninvolved other bed of the same vessel or the opposite cerebral artery. |

[**]Adapted from Higashida et al. Stroke 2003;34:e109–37

**Table A.3** National Institute of Health Stroke Scale

NIH Stroke Scale

| Instructions | Scale definition | Score |
|---|---|---|
| 1a. *Level of consciousness*: The investigator must choose a response, even if a full evaluation is prevented by such obstacles as an endotracheal tube, language barrier, orotracheal trauma/bandages. A 3 is scored only if the patient makes no movement (other than reflexive posturing) in response to noxious stimulation. | 0 = Alert: keenly responsive. <br> 1 = Not alert, but arousable by minor stimulation to obey, answer, or respond. <br> 2 = Not alert, requires repeated stimulation to attend, or is obtunded and requires strong or painful stimulation to make movements (not stereotyped). <br> 3 = Responds only with reflex motor autonomic effects or totally unresponsive, flaccid, and flexic. | —— |
| 1b. *LOC questions*: The patient is asked the month and his/her age. The answer must be correct – there is no partial credit for being close. Aphasic and stuporous patients who do not comprehend the questions will score 2. Patients unable to speak because of endotracheal intubation, orotracheal trauma, severe dysarthria from any cause, language barrier, or any other problem not secondary to aphasia are given a 1. It is important that only the initial answer be graded and that the examiner not "help" the patient with verbal or non-verbal cues. | 0 = Answers both questions correctly. <br> 1 = Answers one question correctly. <br> 2 = Answers neither question correctly. | —— |
| 1c. *LOC commands*: The patient is asked to open and close the eyes and then to grip and release the non-paretic hand. Substitute another one step command if the hands cannot be used. Credit is given if an unequivocal attempt is made but not completed due to weakness. If the patient does not respond to command, the task should be demonstrated to him/her (pantomime) and score the result (i.e., follows none, one or two commands). Patients with trauma, amputation, or other physical impediments should be given suitable one-step commands. Only the first attempt is scored. | 0 = Performs both tasks correctly. <br> 1 = Performs one task correctly. <br> 2 = Performs neither task correctly. | —— |

| | |
|---|---|
| 2. *Best gaze*: Only horizontal eye movements will be tested. Voluntary or reflexive (oculocephalic) eye movements will be scored but caloric testing is not done. If the patient has a conjugate deviation of the eyes that can be overcome by voluntary or reflexive activity, the score will be 1. If a patient has an isolated peripheral nerve paresis (CN III, IV, or VI) score a 1. Gaze is testable in all aphasic patients. Patients with ocular trauma, bandages, pre-existing blindness, or other disorder of visual acuity or fields should be tested with reflexive movements and a choice made by the investigator. Establishing eye contact and then moving about the patient from side to side will occasionally clarify the presence of a partial gaze palsy. | 0 = Normal. <br> 1 = Partial gaze palsy; gaze is abnormal in one or both eyes, but forced deviation or total gaze paresis is not present. <br> 2 = Forced deviation, or total gaze paresis not overcome by the oculocephalic maneuver. |
| 3. *Visual*: Visual fields (upper and lower quadrants) are tested by confrontation, using finger counting or visual threat as appropriate. Patient may be encouraged, but if they look at the side of the moving fingers appropriately, this can be scored as normal. If there is unilateral blindness or enucleation, visual fields in the remaining eye are scored. Score 1 only if a clear-cut asymmetry, including quadrantanopia is found. If patient is blind from any cause, score 3. Double simultaneous stimulation is performed at this point. If there is extinction, patient receives a 1, and the results are used to answer item 11. | 0 = No visual loss. <br> 1 = Partial hemianopia. <br> 2 = Complete hemianopia. <br> 3 = Bilateral hemianopia (blind including cortical blindness). |
| 4. *Facial palsy*: Ask, or use pantomime to encourage the patient to show teeth or raise eyebrows and close eyes. Score symmetry of grimace in response to noxious stimuli in the poorly responsive or non-comprehending patient. If facial trauma/bandages, orotracheal tube, tape, or other physical barrier obscures the face, these should be removed to the extent possible. | 0 = Normal symmetrical movement. <br> 1 = Minor paralysis (flattened nasolabial fold, asymmetry on smiling). <br> 2 = Partial paralysis (total or near total paralysis of lower face). <br> 3 = Complete paralysis of one or both sides (absence of facial movement in the upper and lower face). |

(continued)

**Table A.3** (continued)

NIH Stroke Scale

| Instructions | Scale definition | Score |
|---|---|---|
| 5. *Motor arm*: The limb is placed in the appropriate position: extend the arms (palms down) 90° (if sitting) or 45° (if supine). Drift is scored if the arm falls before 10 s. The aphasic patient is encouraged using urgency in the voice and pantomime, but not noxious stimulation. Each limb is tested in turn, beginning with the non-paretic arm. Only in the case of amputation or joint fusion at the shoulder, the examiner should record the score as untestable (UN), and clearly write the explanation for this choice. | 0 = No drift; limb holds 90° (or 45°) for full 10 s.<br>1 = Drift; limb holds 90° (or 45°), but drifts down before full 10 s: does not hit bed or other support.<br>2 = Some effort against gravity; limb cannot get to or maintain (if cued) 90° (or 45°), drifts down to bed, but has some effort against gravity.<br>3 = No effort against gravity; limb falls.<br>4 = No movement.<br>UN = Amputation or joint fusion, explain: ____<br>5a. *Left arm*<br>5b. *Right arm* | ___<br>___ |
| 6. *Motor leg*: The limb is placed in the appropriate position: hold the leg at 30° (always tested supine). Drift is scored if the leg falls before 5 s. The aphasic patient is encouraged using urgency in the voice and pantomime, but not noxious stimulation. Each limb is tested in turn, beginning with the non-paretic leg. Only in the case of amputation or joint fusion at the hip, the examiner should record the score as untestable (UN), and clearly write the explanation for this choice. | 0 = No drift; leg holds 30-degree position for full 5 s<br>1 = Drift; leg falls by the end of the 5 s period but does not hit bed<br>2 = Some effort against gravity; leg falls to bed by 5 s, but has some effort against gravity<br>3 = No effort against gravity; leg falls to bed immediately<br>4 = No movement<br>UN = Amputation or joint fusion, explain: ____<br>6a. *Left leg*<br>6b. *Right leg* | ___<br>___ |

| 7. *Limb ataxia*: This item is aimed at finding evidence of a unilateral cerebellar lesion. Test with eyes open. In case of visual defect, ensure testing is done in intact visual field. The finger–nose–finger and heel–shin tests are performed on both sides, and ataxia is scored only if present out of proportion to weakness. Ataxia is absent in the patient who cannot understand or is paralyzed. Only in the case of amputation or joint fusion may the item be scored "UN" and the examiner must clearly write the explanation for not scoring. In case of blindness test by touching nose from extended arm position. | 0 = Absent. <br> 1 = Present in one limb. <br> 2 = Present in two limbs. <br> UN = Amputation or joint fusion, explain: _____ | _____ |
| 8. *Sensory*: Sensation or grimace to pinprick when tested, or withdrawal from noxious stimulus in the obtunded or aphasic patient. Only sensory loss attributed to stroke is scored as abnormal and the examiner should test as many body areas [arms (not hands), legs, trunk, face] as needed to accurately check for hemisensory loss. A score of 2, "severe or total sensory loss," should only be given when a severe or total loss of sensation can be clearly demonstrated. Stuporous and aphasic patients will therefore probably score 1 or 0. The patient with brainstem stroke who has bilateral loss of sensation is scored 2. If the patient does not respond and is quadriplegic score 2. Patients in coma (item 1a = 3) are automatically given a 2 on this item. | 0 = Normal; no sensory loss. <br> 1 = Mild to moderate sensory loss; patient feels pinprick is less sharp or is dull on the affected side; or there is a loss of superficial pain with pinprick but patient is aware he/she is being touched. <br> 2 = Severe to total sensory loss; patient is not aware of being touched in the face, arm, and leg. | _____ |

(continued)

**Table A.3** (continued)

NIH Stroke Scale

| Instructions | Scale definition | Score |
|---|---|---|
| 9. *Best language*: A great deal of information about comprehension will be obtained during the preceding sections of the examination. The patient is asked to describe what is happening in the attached picture, to name the items on the attached naming sheet, and to read from the attached list of sentences. Comprehension is judged from responses here as well as to all of the commands in the preceding general neurological exam. If visual loss interferes with the tests, ask the patient to identify objects placed in the hand, repeat, and produce speech. The intubated patient should be asked to write. The patient in coma (item 1a = 3) will automatically score 3 on this item. The examiner must choose a score for the patient with stupor or limited cooperation, but a score of 3 should be used only if the patient is mute and follows no one-step commands. | 0 = No aphasia, normal.<br><br>1 = Mild to moderate aphasia; some obvious loss of fluency or facility of comprehension, without significant limitation on ideas expressed or form of expression. Reduction of speech and/or comprehension, however, makes conversation about provided material difficult or impossible. For example, in conversation about provided materials, examiner can identify picture or naming card content from patient's response.<br><br>2 = Severe aphasia; all communication is through fragmentary expression; great need for inference, questioning, and guessing by the listener. Range of information that can be exchanged is limited; listener carries burden of communication. Examiner cannot identify materials provided from patient response.<br><br>3 = Mute, global aphasia; no usable speech or auditory comprehension. | ___ |
| 10. *Dysarthria*: If patient is thought to be normal, an adequate sample of speech must be obtained by asking patient to read or repeat words from the attached list. If the patient has severe aphasia, the clarity of articulation of spontaneous speech can be rated. Only if the patient is intubated or has other physical barriers to producing speech may the item be scored as untestable (UN), and clearly write an explanation for this choice. Do not tell the patient why he or she is being tested. | 0 = Normal.<br><br>1 = Mild to moderate dysarthria; patient slurs at least some words and, at worst, can be understood with some difficulty.<br><br>2 = Severe; patient's speech is so slurred as to be unintelligible in the absence of or out of proportion to any dysphasia, or is mute/anarthric.<br><br>3 = Intubated or other physical barrier, explain: | ___ |

11. *Extinction and inattention (formerly neglect)*: Sufficient information to identify neglect may be obtained during the prior testing. If the patient has a severe visual loss preventing visual double simultaneous stimulation, and the cutaneous stimuli are normal, the score is normal. If the patient has aphasia but does appear to attend to both sides, the score is normal. The presence of visual spatial neglect or anosagnosia may also be taken as evidence of abnormality. Since the abnormality is scored only if present, the item is never untestable.

0 = Normal abnormality.

1 = Visual, tactile, auditory, spatial, or personal inattention or extinction to bilateral simultaneous stimulation in one of the sensory modalities.

2 = Profound hemi-inattention or extinction to more than one modality; does not recognize own hand or orients to only one side of space.

**Table A.3.1**  Modified Rankin Scale

0. No symptoms at all
1. No significant disability despite symptoms: able to carry out all usual duties and activities
2. Slight disability: unable to carry out all previous activities, but able to look after own affairs without assistance
3. Moderate disability: requiring some help, but able to walk without assistance
4. Moderately severe disability: unable to walk without assistance, and unable to attend to own bodily needs without assistance
5. Severe disability: bedridden, incontinent, and requiring constant nursing care and attention
6. Dead

**Table A.3.2**  Barthel Index

| | |
|---|---|
| Feeding | 0 = Unable |
| | 5 = Needs help cutting, spreading butter, etc., or requires modified diet |
| | 10 = Independent |
| Bathing | 0 = Dependent |
| | 5 = Independent (or in shower) |
| Grooming | 0 = Needs help with personal care |
| | 5 = Independent face/hair/teeth/shaving (implements provided) |
| Dressing | 0 = Dependent |
| | 5 = Needs help but can do about half unaided |
| | 10 = Independent (including buttons, zips, laces, etc.) |
| Bowels | 0 = Incontinent (or needs to be given enemas) |
| | 5 = Occasional accident |
| | 10 = Continent |
| Bladder | 0 = Incontinent, or catheterized and unable to manage alone |
| | 5 = Occasional accident |
| | 10 = Continent |
| Toilet use | 0 = Dependent |
| | 5 = Needs some help, but can do something alone |
| | 10 = Independent (on and off, dressing, wiping) |
| Transfers bed to chair and back | 0 = Unable, no sitting balance |
| | 5 = Major help (one or two people, physical), can sit |
| | 10 = Minor help (verbal or physical) |
| | 15 = Independent |
| Mobility | 0 = Immobile or <50 yards |
| | 5 = Wheelchair independent, including corners, >50 yards |
| | 10 = Walks with help of one person (verbal or physical) >50 yards |
| | 15 = Independent (but may use any aid; for example, stick) >50 yards |
| Stairs | 0 = Unable |
| | 5 = Needs help (verbal, physical, carrying aid) |
| | 10 = Independent |

**Table A.4** Cincinnati Pre-hospital Stroke Scale

| Facial droop | Normal: both sides of face move equally |
| | Abnormal: one side of face does not move at all |
| Arm drift | Normal: both arms move equally or not at all |
| | Abnormal: one arm drifts compared to the other |
| Speech | Normal: patient uses correct words with no slurring |
| | Abnormal: slurred or inappropriate words or mute |

Kothari et al. (1999)

**Table A.5** FAST Stroke Scale

| Facial weakness | Can the person smile? Has their mouth or eye drooped? |
| Arm weakness | Can the person raise both arms? |
| Speech problems | Can the person speak clearly and understand what you say? |
| Time | Time to call 999 |

http://www.dh.gov.uk/en/Publicationsandstatistics/Publications/PublicationsPolicyAnd
Guidance/DH_094239, last accessed 18.10.11

# Reference

Kothari RU, Pancioli A, Liu T, Brott T, Broderick J (1999) Cincinnati Pre-hospital Stroke
    Scale: reproducibility and validity. Ann Emerg Med 33(4):373–378

# Index

I.Q. Grunwald et al., *How to set up an Acute Stroke Service*,
DOI 10.1007/978-3-642-21405-9, © Springer-Verlag Berlin Heidelberg 2012

Printing: Ten Brink, Meppel, The Netherlands
Binding: Stürtz, Würzburg, Germany